HIV/AIDS NURSING CARE PLANS

2nd edition

Lucy Bradley-Springer, Ph.D., R.N., A.C.R.N.

Assistant Professor
University of New Mexico,
School of Medicine

Co-Director
New Mexico AIDS Education and Training Center
University of New Mexico School of Medicine,
Albuquerque, New Mexico

Skidmore-Roth Publishing, Inc.

PUBLISHING

Publisher: Linda Skidmore-Roth
Cover Design: Angel J. Lopez
Developmental Editors: Molly Sullivan, Rae Robertson
Copy Editor: Kathryn Head, B.A.
Typesetter: Gary Grudowski

Notice: The author and publisher of this volume have taken care to make certain that all information is correct and compatible with standards generally accepted at the time of publication. Because the science of nursing is constantly changing and expanding, new techniques and concepts are continually implemented. Therefore, the reader is encouraged to stay abreast of new developments in the nursing field and to be aware that policies vary according to the guidelines of each school or institution.

Bradley-Springer, Lucy
AIDS Nursing Care Plans—2nd edition

ISBN 1-56930-097-6
1. Nursing-Handbooks, Manuals
2. Medical-Handbooks, Manuals

SKIDMORE-ROTH PUBLISHING, INC.
400 Inverness Drive South, Suite 260
Englewood, CO 80112
1-800-825-3150
www.skidmore-roth.com

Consultants

Heather Andersen, R.N., M.N.
Psychosocial/Mental Health Curriculum
and Training Specialist
AIDS Education and Training Center
University of Washington
Seattle, Washington

Debra K. Brown, R.N., B.S.N., O.C.N.
HIV Nurse Coordinator
AIDS Education Training Center (ETC) Coordinator
University of Nebraska Medical Center
Omaha, Nebraska

Ruth M. Neil, R.N., Ph.D.
Project Director
Denver Nursing Project in Human Caring
Assistant Professor
University of Colorado, School of Nursing
Denver, Colorado

Introductory Remarks

One thing you can say about HIV infection is that there is never a dull moment. Ten years ago when I started working in this field we had very little to work with: a test, a drug, and a lot of hope. Three years ago when I started working on the first edition of this book, we had made many advances but I was already aware that major changes were on the way. In the past three years we have learned a lot about HIV and how it affects the human immune system. Approved drugs expanded from four drugs in a single class to 12 drugs in three classes, and many more drugs are in various stages of development. Advances have been made in other areas, too: assessing the extent of disease, treating opportunistic diseases, and helping people live with HIV as a chronic disease. Doing the revisions on this book has reinforced for me the rapidity with which science can move. It has also reinforced for me the bitter facts of this epidemic: a continuous supply of newly infected individuals, predominantly among people with fewer and fewer resources; no vaccine; continued reticence on the part of leaders to take the hard political stands needed to encourage prevention; treatments that are not available or effective for many; unabated stigma and discrimination; and the absence of a cure.

During the past ten years I have depended upon many people for support and encouragement. I have been inspired by nurses I have known in New Mexico and across the country through my associations with the Mountain-Plains Regional AIDS Education and Training Center and the Association of Nurses in AIDS Care. These men and women have amazed me with their perseverance in the face of severe adversity, with their competence in the face of ignorance, and with their caring in the face of overwhelming odds.

Their work has in no small way contributed to the advances that have been made in this field. Some of those nurses are no longer with us, but their impact is felt everyday in clinics and hospitals and the homes of HIV-infected clients. This book is for those nurses and I only hope that it in some way honors their efforts.

This book is also for the clients that all nurses work with—HIV infected or not. I hope it emphasizes the need for prevention at all levels, especially in primary care. We have not yet learned important lessons about sexuality, drug use, violence, racism, sexism, classism, and discrimination that should have been learned long ago. HIV is a consequence of not having learned those lessons; it is also an opportunity to figure out these problems and to progress to a state where we do not have to fear the next tragic epidemic. Nurses have a responsibility to lead the way in this revolution and we must advance for our own sakes as well as the sakes of those we love.

Revising this book has also reinforced the importance of family for me. The book reflects this fact for clients and nurses, but I must be clear in the debt I owe to my own family for the assistance they have afforded me throughout the years and especially during the times when I become immersed in writing projects. My husband, Bob Springer, exhibits patience and support during long writing sessions as do my parents and siblings. And, as always, I cannot finish a major project without honoring the memory of my father, George H. Bradley, Jr., who always encouraged me to do more and to do it better.

Lucy Bradley-Springer

Table of Contents

Chapter I

Introduction

In 1981, public health officials in the United States recognized a new disease that eventually became known as the acquired immunodeficiency syndrome (AIDS). We now know that AIDS is the final phase of a progressive immune function disorder caused by the human immunodeficiency virus (HIV). The following statistics for HIV infection and AIDS show the extent of the epidemic in the United States and its territories. By the end of 1997, over 641,000 cases of AIDS had been diagnosed and over 390,000 AIDS-related deaths had been reported (Centers for Disease Control and Prevention [CDC], 1998). In 1995, HIV infection was the fourth leading cause of years of productive life lost (Selik & Chu, 1997). An estimated 650,000 to 900,000 people are infected with HIV and the fastest growing groups of people with HIV are women and adolescents (Ungvarski, 1997). In addition, 10% of people with AIDS in the United States are 50 years of age or older (Whipple & Scura, 1996). AIDS is not only changing along the lines of gender and age, it is also becoming an increasing problem for people of color, people who live in poverty, people who live in rural areas (Ungvarski, 1997), and people who deal with violence in their lives (Seals, 1996).

Globally, HIV is even more devastating. In 1997, 5.8 million people were newly infected with HIV, including 3.1 million men, 2.1 million women, and 590,000 children. An estimated 30.6 million people with HIV infection were living in the world in December of 1997. The United Nations AIDS Project estimates that 16,000 new cases of the infection occur every day. It is further estimated that 1 in every 100 adults in the world is infected with HIV and that 90% of these people are unaware of their infections. AIDS has killed 11.7 million people since the beginning of the pandemic and produced 8.2 million uninfected orphans whose mothers died of the disease. By the year 2000, an estimated 40 million people will have been infected with HIV (Joint United Nations Programme, 1997).

There is good news, however, especially for those who live in the United States, Western Europe, Canada, and Australia. Since 1994, several important advances have been made: the development of laboratory tests to assess viral levels in the blood; the production of new groups of antiretroviral agents; multi-drug therapy; treatment to decrease the risk of perinatal transmission (Ungvarski, 1997); and improved protocols for those exposed to HIV infection at work (Porche, 1997). These important advances have made it possible to improve the quality and quantity of life for many people living with HIV disease and to decrease the risks of those who come into contact with them. Unfortunately, these advances are not universally effective or available for all of those who need them, even in the developed countries. Although great progress has been made, the HIV epidemic is not over and nursing care continues to be a critical need.

Pathophysiology of HIV Infection

HIV is an RNA virus that was discovered in 1983 (see Figure 1.1). RNA viruses are called retroviruses because they replicate in a "backward" manner (going from RNA to DNA). Like all viruses, HIV is an obligate parasite: It cannot survive and replicate unless it is inside a living cell. HIV enters a cell through a series of complex chemical and physical actions (McNicholl, Smith, Qari, & Hodge, 1997) when the gp120 "knobs" on the viral envelope bind to specific (CD4) receptor sites on the cell's surface (see Figure 1.2). Cells with CD4 receptor sites on their surfaces, including lymphocytes, macrophages, monocytes, follicular

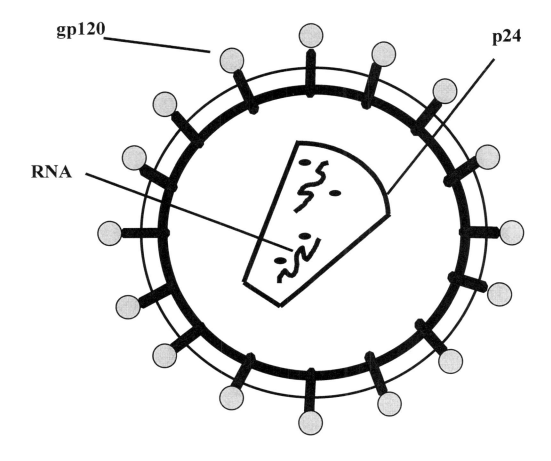

Figure 1.1. The Human Immunodeficiency Virus (HIV). HIV is a retrovirus that is surrounded by an envelope made up of proteins (including gp120). HIV contains a core of viral RNA and proteins (including p24). HIV makes a variety of enzymes, including reverse transcriptase (RT), that are necessary for viral replication.

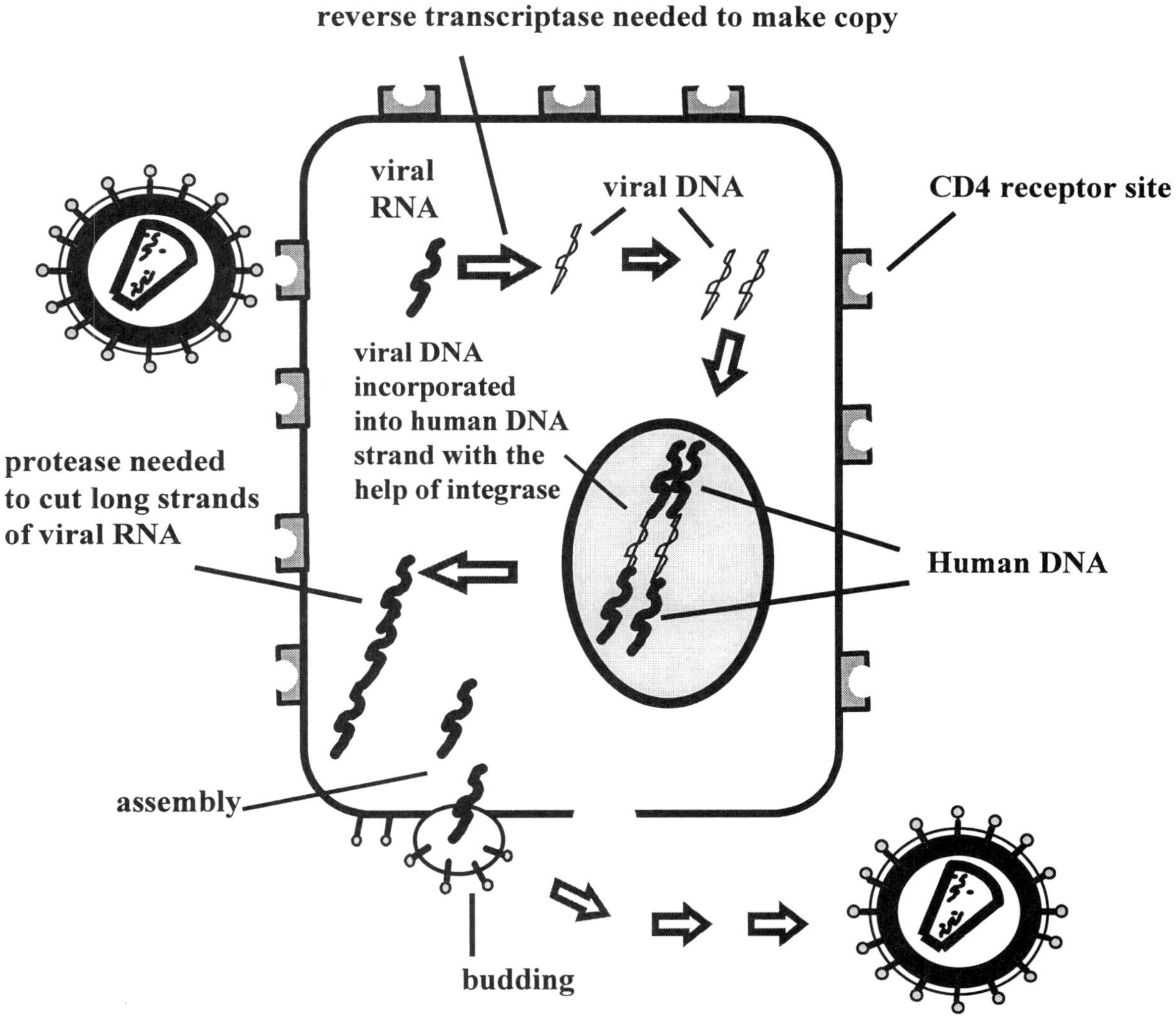

Figure 1.2. HIV Replication. Viral gp120 proteins attach to CD4 receptor sites on the cell membrane through a series of mechanical and chemical processes. Viral RNA enters the cell and, in the presence of reverse transcriptase, makes double stranded viral DNA. The viral DNA incorporates itself into the cellular genome with the assistance of integrase, causing permanent cellular infection and directing the production of new viruses. Viral replication includes the production of long strands of viral RNA that must be cut to the appropriate lengths in order to survive. This is accomplished with the assistance of protease. Newly formed viruses then bud out from the membrane of the infected cell, taking a bit of the cell's membrane to form the new viral envelope.

dendritic cells (FDCs), and some cells in the nervous system, are at risk of becoming infected through this process (Brennan & Porche, 1997).

Once bound, the virus is internalized in the cell and its genetic material is uncoated. There, with the assistance of an enzyme called reverse transcriptase, viral RNA is transcribed into a single strand of viral DNA. The DNA strand replicates itself, becoming double stranded viral DNA. At this point, viral DNA can enter the cell's nucleus and, with the assistance of an enzyme called integrase, splice itself into the genome, becoming a permanent part of the cell's genetic structure. Viral replication continues when viral DNA directs the cell to make more HIV. Production of HIV within the cell is a complex process, resulting in long strands of HIV RNA that must be cut into appropriate lengths. Cleaving of these genetic strands, accomplished with the assistance of the enzyme protease, is necessary for the production of mature, viable, and infectious HIV (Brennan & Porche, 1997; Greene, 1997; Lisanti & Zwolski, 1997). Within a few days of infection, viral replication is established and progresses at a steady and rapid rate. As many as 10 billion new HIV particles can be produced on a daily basis in HIV-infected individuals (Ho et al., 1995). The rapidity with which HIV replicates is problematic. Not only does it provide a constant source of virions to maintain the active infection, it also enhances the risk of replication errors that result in the viral mutations that cause difficulties in vaccine development and lead to drug resistance (Haynes, 1996; Mellors, 1996; Ungvarski, 1997).

Although HIV can infect several types of human cells, immune dysfunction results predominantly from the destruction of T-helper cells, more appropriately called CD4+ T lymphocytes. Remember that

T-helper cells play a pivotal role in the human immune response. They recognize problems (such as cancer cells and invading infectious organisms) and then secrete cytokines (chemicals) that initiate the body's immune defenses. CD4+ T lymphocytes are targeted by HIV because they have more CD4 receptor sites on their surfaces than other CD4 bearing cells.

The normal life span of a CD4+ T lymphocyte is 100 days, but HIV-infected cells die after an average life span of only two days. Viral activity destroys about one billion CD4+ T lymphocytes every day. Fortunately, the bone marrow and thymus are able, for a number of years, to produce enough CD4+ T lymphocytes to replace those that have been destroyed. The result is the maintenance of a steady-state viral load/CD4+ T lymphocyte count. Eventually, however, the ability of HIV to destroy CD4+ T lymphocytes exceeds the capability to replace the cells, and the result is an increase in the viral load, a decline in the CD4+ T lymphocyte count, and a concomitant decrease in immune capability. HIV can kill CD4+ T lymphocytes in a number of ways including disruption of cellular structure and function; fusion of infected cells into large, multi-nucleated, nonviable cells (syncytia); and host immune responses (Brennan & Porche, 1997). The ultimate result is that so many CD4+ T lymphocytes are destroyed that normal immune function does not occur and the coordination of immune responses suffers (Staprans & Feinberg, 1997). This sets the stage for the development of life-threatening opportunistic diseases.

Initial infection with HIV causes a decrease in the number of CD4+ T lymphocytes in the presence of HIV viremia (see Figure 1.3). Fluctuations in CD4+ T cells and viral quantities are seen for several months after the initial infection until stabilization is reached.

Stabilization results in a "set point," or baseline viral load, that is maintained during the prolonged period of asymptomatic disease. It is clear that those individuals with a high viral set point progress more rapidly in their disease than those with a lower set point (Feinberg, 1996). One study found that individuals with RNA levels of greater than 100,000 copies/mm³ within six months of infection increased the risk of progression to AIDS within five years ten times above those whose viral loads stayed below 100,000 copies/mm³ (Jones & Gelone, 1997).

In a normal immune response, foreign antigens filter through lymph tissue where they are trapped by the follicular dendritic cell (FDC) network and presented directly to B cells and T lymphocytes. In the initial stages of HIV infection, these cells respond and function normally. B cells make

HIV-specific antibody that helps to reduce viral loads in the blood (see Figure 1.3). The T-helper cells that respond to the site of viruses trapped in the lymph nodes are activated to initiate the cellular immune response. These activated cells provide an ideal target for HIV. They are attracted to the site of concentrated HIV where they are exposed to infection through viral contact with the CD4 receptor sites. Once infected, activated cells support viral replication and assist in spreading or seeding the infection throughout the lymph system. Lymphoid tissue thus becomes an early reservoir for HIV, promoting active replication even during periods of clinical latency. Eventually, HIV causes significant degenerative changes to the FDC network. This is an important development because it allows viral particles to spill over into the blood (a factor in disease progression) and it represents

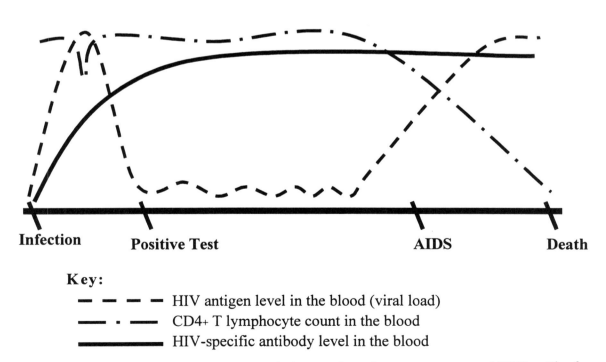

Key:

    − − − −   HIV antigen level in the blood (viral load)
    —— · ——   CD4+ T lymphocyte count in the blood
    ————   HIV-specific antibody level in the blood

Figure 1.3. Markers. Viral load in the blood, CD4+ T lymphocyte counts, and HIV antibody levels over the spectrum of HIV infection.

significant impairment of the immune system's ability to respond to new infections (Lisanti & Zwolski, 1997).

Detecting HIV Infection

The most useful screening tests for HIV are those that detect HIV-specific antibody. The major problem with these tests is the delay of 3 weeks to 6 months before detectable antibody is produced (see Figures 1.3 and 1.4). This creates a "window period" during which an infected individual will not test HIV antibody positive. The following steps are used in the process of testing blood for antibodies to HIV:

1. A highly sensitive enzyme immunoassay (EIA, ELISA) is done to detect serum antibodies that bind to HIV antigens on test plates. Blood samples that are negative on this test are reported as negative.
2. If the blood is EIA reactive, the test is repeated.
3. If the blood is repeatedly EIA reactive, a more specific confirming test such as the Western blot (WB) or immunofluorescence assay (IFA) is done.

- WB testing uses purified HIV antigen electrophoresed on gels; these are incubated with serum samples. If antibody in the serum is present, it can be detected.
- IFA is used to identify HIV in infected cells. Blood is treated with a fluorescent antibody against viral proteins and then examined using a fluorescent microscope.
4. Blood that is reactive in all of the first three steps is reported as HIV-antibody positive.
5. If the results are indeterminant, testing should be repeated at a later date. Consistently indeterminant test results require the use of polymerase chain reaction (PCR), viral culture, or other diagnostic measures.
   - PCR analyzes DNA extracted from lymphocytes and/or HIV from serum using an *in vitro* amplification procedure.
   - A cell culture system can be used to grow viruses from infected lymphocytes.

Because these tests are expensive and difficult to do, they are not used for

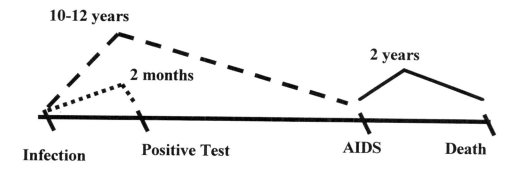

Figure 1.4. Timeline for HIV Disease Progression. Median times between points in HIV disease progression.

screening purposes, but may be done in situations where the index of suspicion is high and antibody tests are negative.

Laboratory Indicators of Disease Progression

The progression of HIV infection has been monitored by CD4+ T lymphocyte counts for many years. As the disease progresses, there is usually a decrease in the number of CD4+ T lymphocytes, a marker for decreased immune function (see Figure 1.3). The normal CD4+ T lymphocyte count for an adult is 800-1200 cells per cubic millimeter (mm³) of blood. Generally, the immune system remains healthy with more than 500 CD4+ T lymphocytes/mm³. Minor immune problems start to occur when the count drops to 200-499 CD4+ T lymphocytes/mm³, and severe problems develop when there are fewer than 200 CD4+ T lymphocytes/mm³. It has been clear, however, that CD4+ T lymphocyte counts, while extremely important, revealed only part of the clinical picture (Bartlett, 1996).

Improved technologies that allow for the quantitation of viral activity have resulted in the ability to better assess clinical status and disease progression. Viral load (also referred to as viral burden or HIV RNA level) quantifies viral particles in a biological sample (usually serum). Viral loads can be determined with quantitative competitive PCR (RT-PCR) and branched-chain DNA (bDNA) techniques (Hughes et al., 1997; O'Brien, Hartigan, Daar, Simberkoff, & Hamilton, 1997; Saag, 1997). Viral load measurements are reported in copies/mm³, and when they are very low, they may be reported as undetectable. This does not mean that there are no viruses in the sample, nor does it mean that the patient is cured; it simply means that the number of viruses in the blood is too small to detect by current tests. High values can range into the hundreds of thousands. Because the numbers are so large, changes in viral loads are reported in log values. While this may be confusing at first, the main thing to remember is that the goal is for the viral load to go down and that a 1 log drop represents a 90% decrease in viral load, a 2 log drop represents a 95% decrease, and a 3 log drop indicates that 99% of the viral load has been eliminated.

Viral load assessments, used in conjunction with information about immune status derived from CD4+ T cell counts, provide an important core of information for evolving treatment protocols. They help to determine when to initiate therapy, define how well treatments are working (or not), and evaluate if clinical goals are being met (Hughes et al., 1997; O'Brien, Hartigan, Daar, Simberkoff, & Hamilton, 1997; Saag, 1997).

Transmission

HIV is a fragile virus that can only be transmitted under specific conditions. It is transmitted from human to human through infected blood, semen, vaginal secretions, and breast milk. If these infected fluids are introduced into an uninfected person's body, there is a potential for transmission. Transmission of HIV has occurred through sexual intercourse with an infected partner, internalized contact with HIV-infected blood or blood products, and perinatal transmission during pregnancy, at the time of delivery, or through breast feeding (Casey, Cohen, & Hughes, 1996; Lisanti & Zwolski, 1997). In addition, transmission has occurred after artificial insemination with HIV-infected semen and through organ transplantations when the donor was HIV infected.

HIV-infected individuals can transmit the virus to others within a few days after initial infection. Ability to transmit HIV is lifelong after that: There is no noninfectious state with HIV. Transmission of HIV is subjected to the same requirements as other organisms: A sufficient amount of the infectious agent must be introduced through an appropriate portal of entry into a susceptible host. Duration and frequency of contact, quantity of inoculant, virulence of the organism, and host immune defense capability all affect whether infection will actually occur after an exposure.

The viral load in the blood, semen, vaginal secretions, or breast milk of the "donor" is an important variable. In HIV infection, large amounts of virus are detected in the blood and semen during the first few months after initial infection and again during the late stages of the disease (see Figure 1.3). Unprotected sexual or blood exposure to an infected individual is more risky during these periods, although HIV can be transmitted during all phases of the disease (Staprans & Feinberg, 1997).

HIV is not spread casually. The virus cannot be transmitted through hugging, kissing, shaking hands, sharing eating utensils or attending school with an HIV-infected person. It cannot be transmitted through sputum, urine, emesis, feces, tears, saliva, or sweat unless those fluids also contain blood. In addition, there is no evidence that the virus can be transmitted by insects (Casey et al., 1996). Repeated studies have failed to demonstrate transmission of the virus by respiratory droplets, enteric routes, or casual encounters in any setting and health care workers have a very low occupational risk of acquiring the virus, even after a needle stick injury ("Health care worker occupational exposure," 1994; Ungvarski, 1997).

Sexual Transmission

Sexual contact with an HIV-infected partner is the most common method of transmission. Sexual activity provides an opportunity for contact with semen, vaginal secretions, and/or blood. Although men who have sex with men (MSM) were the initial targets of HIV in North American and Western Europe, heterosexual transmission is becoming more prevalent; it is now the most common method of infection for women in the United States, causing 40% of all AIDS cases in women from July 1996 through June 1997 (CDC, 1998). The most important variable is whether HIV is present in one of the sexual partners, not whether the couple is homosexual or heterosexual.

The most risky form of sexual intercourse is unprotected receptive anal intercourse. While many people associate anal intercourse exclusively with MSM, remember that many heterosexual couples also use this form of sexual expression. Forceful anal or vaginal intercourse may result in trauma to mucosal surfaces. This increases the likelihood of infection with HIV (and all other sexually transmitted diseases [STDs]) because tearing of the mucous membrane provides a portal of entry for the virus.

During any form of sexual intercourse (anal, vaginal, or oral), the risk of infection is considerably greater for the receptive partner (the one who "receives" the semen), although infection can also be transmitted to an inserting partner (the one who "deposits" the semen). The receiver's increased risk is related to his/her prolonged contact with the semen. This may contribute to the fact that women are more easily infected than men during heterosexual intercourse (Staprans & Feinberg, 1997). A large number of different sexual partners have been associated with HIV infection in the past, but increasing prevalence rates make this less of a factor. Sexual intercourse with one partner who is HIV-infected creates a risk while sexual intercourse with a lot of uninfected partners results in no risk for HIV infection.

Contact with Blood and Blood Products

HIV is transmitted by exposure to contaminated blood through the accidental or intended sharing of injection equipment. Sharing equipment to inject illicit drugs is a major means of transmission to both sexes in many large metropolitan areas and is becoming more common in smaller cities and rural areas. It is important to remember, however, that equipment used to inject drugs such as insulin, vitamin B_{12}, clotting factor, steroids, and amphetamines is also contaminated after use. It doesn't matter what has been injected: Used equipment is potentially contaminated and should not be shared (Casey et al., 1996).

In 1985, routine screening of blood donors to identify individuals at high risk and testing donated blood for the presence of HIV antibody was implemented in the United States and other developed countries, improving the safety of the blood supply. In those countries where blood is routinely tested, HIV infection as a result of blood transfusions is now unlikely, but still possible because blood donated during the window period will not show HIV-specific antibody on testing (Masci, 1996). No new cases of HIV related to the use of clotting factor are expected because these products are now treated with heat or chemicals to kill the virus (Flaskerud, 1995a).

By the end of 1997, 54 health care workers in the United States were shown to have been infected with HIV through occupational exposure and the CDC was following 132 more who may have been infected at work; of these, the largest proportion (30%) were nurses (CDC, 1998). HIV can be occupationally transmitted during exposure to HIV-infected fluids through percutaneous injury and nonintact skin and mucous membranes. The greatest risk for occupational transmission of HIV occurs through puncture wounds. The risk of infection after a needle stick exposure to HIV-infected blood is 0.3% to 0.4%. The risk is higher if the exposure is caused by blood from a patient with a high viral load; if the puncture wound is deep; if the needle is hollow bore with visible blood; if the device had provided venous or arterial access; or if the patient dies within 60 days of the exposure. Splash exposures of blood to skin with an open lesion also present some risk, although the risk is much lower than from a puncture wound (CDC, 1996; Porche, 1997; Ungvarski, 1997).

Perinatal Transmission

Among children with AIDS in the United States who are less than 13 years of age, 91% were infected at birth (CDC, 1998). Transmission from an HIV-infected mother to her infant can occur during pregnancy, at the time of delivery, or after birth through breast feeding (Mandelbrot, 1997). Studies in various countries have found that 14-45% of infants born to HIV-infected women will be born with HIV (Flaskerud, 1995a); this means that 55-86% of these infants will not be infected. A study in Kenshasa, Zaire found that infants whose HIV-infected mothers did not demonstrate specific markers for immune deficiency had only a 7% rate of infection while those whose mothers showed significant immune dysfunction were infected 71% of the time (St. Louis et al., 1993), indicating that transmission risks increase with advancing disease in the mother. In addition, emerging data about the outcomes of perinatally infected children show that most of these children live longer than initially expected. One longitudinal study of 529 perinatally infected children found a median survival time of 96.2 months with 49.5% still living at age nine (Tovo et al., 1992). This information is helpful when counseling HIV-infected people who are struggling with difficult decisions related to reproduction (Bradley-Springer, 1994).

Diagnosis of HIV in infants can be problematic. All infants born to HIV-infected mothers test positive for HIV antibody because maternal HIV antibody crosses the placental barrier and remains present in the infant for up to 18 months. For that reason, early detection of HIV infection in infants depends on testing for HIV antigen through the use of PCR or viral culture; these tests can definitively diagnose HIV in infected infants by four weeks of age (Casey et al., 1996).

Preventing Transmission of HIV

Public health measures to decrease the risk of transmission of infectious diseases hinge on two tactics: vaccination and behavior modification. Both of these are factors in the HIV epidemic.

HIV Vaccine

Early in the epidemic, there was optimism that an HIV vaccine would be quickly developed (Caldwell, 1993). Despite considerable research and development, a vaccine still eludes scientists and there is no hope for an effective preventive vaccine within the near future (Johnston, 1997). The problems that inhibit vaccine development are numerous. HIV is an intracellular pathogen: It can hide from circulating immune factors. HIV

is highly variable: It mutates rapidly so that infected individuals develop a number of HIV variants that may not all respond to a simple vaccine. This is compounded by the fact that two strains of HIV (HIV-1 and HIV-2) cause AIDS and at least ten clades (or families) of HIV-1 exist around the world (Ungvarski, 1997). Development of an effective vaccine for Clade B (the predominant group in the Americas and Western Europe) may not prove effective in developing countries where the need is even greater (Johnston, 1997). A further issue in HIV vaccine development is that the indicators of protective immunity for HIV are unknown: Antibody development after vaccination usually indicates immunity, but HIV-infected clients produce an antibody that does not prevent active infection or confer immunity (Haynes, 1996). In addition, HIV is frequently transmitted through mucosal routes: A successful vaccine would need to induce mucosal as well as systemic protection (Grady & Kelly, 1996; Mascola, McNeil, & Burke, 1994).

There are also social, ethical, and economic issues associated with the development of an HIV vaccine. A major problem is related to the fact that there is no adequate animal model for HIV. Vaccine efficacy can, therefore, be established only through human testing. Even when volunteers are recruited for the research trials, there are problems related to the possibility of accidental infection and the difficulty of establishing vaccine effectiveness (Grady & Kelly, 1996; Johnston, 1997). Unlike other viruses for which vaccines exist, the development of HIV antibody will not necessarily result in protection from HIV.

Despite the difficult nature of these problems, considerable HIV vaccine research is in progress. Several vaccines are in development and a few have progressed to human trials (Grady & Kelly, 1996). Investigations are also progressing on vaccines that boost HIV-specific host immune responses for use in already infected clients. Authorities warn, however, that the development of a successful vaccine will not replace current prevention methods based on education and behavior change because no vaccine is likely to be 100% effective (Johnston, 1997).

Protective Behaviors

Even without a vaccine, HIV transmission and new cases of HIV are preventable. Specific protective behaviors have been known and recommended since the mid-1980s. These behaviors are crucial for control of the epidemic. Prevention techniques can be divided into SAFE activities (those that eliminate risk) and RISK REDUCING activities (those that decrease, but do not eliminate, risk). HIGH RISK behaviors occur when no effective efforts are taken to control or eliminate risk (see Table 1.1). Harm reduction measures encourage clients to adopt behaviors that are safer, healthier, or less risky than their current behaviors in order to improve health and decrease risks. While this sounds simple, it isn't. The major reason that it isn't simple is that we are dealing with people and trying to get them to change behaviors that have meaning or value or history or are simply more convenient and comfortable than the behaviors that will provide protection. With this in mind, the following section discusses primary prevention tactics for HIV infection.

Decreasing Risks Related to Sexual Intercourse

Safe activities eliminate the risk of exposure to HIV in semen and vaginal secretions. Abstaining from all sexual activity is the most effective way to accomplish this goal. There are, however, safe options for those

who do not wish to abstain. Outercourse, or limiting sexual behavior to activities in which the mouth, penis, vagina, or rectum does not come into contact with the partner's mouth, penis, vagina, or rectum, is safe because there is no contact with blood, semen, or vaginal secretions. Safe activities include massage, masturbation, mutual masturbation (hand jobs), telephone sex, or other activities that meet the "no contact" requirements. Insertive sex is considered to be safe only in a mutually monogamous relationship with a partner who is not infected with HIV or at risk of becoming infected with HIV. The problem with mutual monogamy is that both partners have to follow all of the rules all of the time. Unfortunately, a number of cases of HIV infection have occurred in individuals who were not aware that their partners had not remained monogamous.

Risk reducing sexual activities decrease the risk of contact with HIV through the use of barriers. Barriers should be used when engaging in sexual activity with a partner whose HIV status is not known or with a partner who is known to be HIV infected. The most commonly used barrier is the male condom. Condoms, when used correctly and consistently, are over 98% effective in preventing the transmission of HIV (Carey et al., 1992; de Vincenzi, 1994; Messiah et al., 1997). Major points for correct use of the male condom include the following:

- Condoms should be made out of good quality latex or polyurethane. "Natural skin" condoms have pores that are large enough for HIV to penetrate and should not be used for disease prevention.
- Condoms should be stored in a cool, dry place, where they are protected from trauma. Friction caused by improper care can wear down the latex.

- A condom should not be used past its expiration date or if the package looks worn or punctured.
- Lubricants used in conjunction with condoms must be water soluble. Oil-based lubricants can weaken latex and increase the risk of tearing or breaking. Non-lubricated condoms (with or without flavors) can provide protection during oral intercourse.
- The condom must be placed on the erect penis before any contact is made with the partner's mouth, vagina, or rectum to prevent exposure to pre-ejaculatory secretions that may contain HIV.
- The penis and condom should be removed from the partner's body immediately after ejaculation and before the erection is lost to prevent fluid from leaking out of the condom around a flaccid penis.
- Condoms are not reusable. They should be discarded after use and a new condom used for every act of intercourse.

Female condoms are now available in most communities and, although more expensive than male condoms, they provide an important option for some couples. Some couples have reported that the female condom feels better than the male condom; others like male condoms better. The only way for clients to find out which type of condom works best for them is to try them both. Use can be complicated, so careful instructions and practice are required. General guidelines for using female condoms include:

- Female condoms consist of a polyurethane sheath with two springform rings. The smaller ring is inserted into the vagina and holds the condom in place internally around the cervix. This ring can be removed if the condom is to be used for anal intercourse. It *should not be removed* if the condom is to be used for vaginal intercourse. The larger ring surrounds the opening to the condom. It functions to keep the condom in place externally while protecting the external genitalia.
- Water soluble lubrication should be used with female condoms. Female condoms come pre-lubricated, but additional lubrication may be needed. Lubrication protects the condom from tearing during sexual intercourse and can also decrease the noise that results from friction of the penis against the condom.
- The client will need to practice inserting the female condom. Lubrication makes the condom slippery and this can be frustrating until skill is gained.
- During sexual intercourse, the penis must be inserted into the female condom through the outer ring. It is possible for the penis to miss this opening, thus making contact with the vagina and defeating the purpose of the condom.
- A male condom should not be used at the same time as a female condom.
- Immediately after intercourse, the condom should be removed before standing up. The outer ring should be twisted to keep the semen inside before gently pulling the condom out of the vagina or rectum.
- Female condoms should be discarded after use and a new condom used for each act of intercourse.

Squares of latex (available from dental supply sources) or plastic wrapping paper can be used to cover the external female genitalia during oral sexual activity. Latex panties, which provide a stabilized covering of the external female genitalia, are now available in some areas.

Decreasing Risks Related to Drug Use

Even before the HIV epidemic, it was pretty clear that drug use is harmful. It can cause immune suppression and malnutrition as well as a host of psychosocial problems, but drug use in and of itself does not cause HIV infection. The major risks for HIV are related to sharing injection equipment and having unsafe sexual experiences while under the influence. The basic rules are: Don't use drugs; If you use, don't share equipment; and Don't have sexual intercourse when under the influence of any drug (including alcohol) that impairs decision-making ability.

The safest mechanism is to abstain from all drug use and this tactic should be encouraged. However, abstinence may not be a viable alternative for users who choose not to quit or for those who have no access to drug treatment services. The risk of HIV for these individuals can be eliminated if they can find alternatives to injecting. Other routes of drug administration such as smoking, snorting, or ingesting are safe because they remove the risk of exposure to blood through injection equipment. Risk can also be eliminated if users do not share their injection equipment. Injection equipment includes needles, syringes, cookers (spoons or bottle caps used to mix the drug), cotton, and rinse water. None of this equipment should be shared.

The safest tactic is for continuing users to have access to sterile equipment. Some communities now support needle and syringe exchange programs (N/SEPs) that provide sterile equipment to users. Opposition to these programs is supported by the fear that ready access to injection supplies will increase drug use (Bradley-Springer,

1997a). Studies have shown, however, that in communities where exchange programs have been established, drug use does not increase and rates of HIV infection are controlled (Des Jarlais, Friedman, Choopanya, Vanichseni, & Ward, 1992; Lurie et al., 1993). Importantly, studies from communities around the world have not found any trends suggesting that N/SEPs increase drug use, the number of new drug users, or inappropriate disposal of contaminated syringes (Lurie et al., 1993; Normand, Vlahov, & Moses, 1995). Instead, N/SEPs are associated with economic and general health benefits. Lurie and Drucker (1996) reported that had wide-spread institution of N/SEPs occurred in the United States in 1987, an estimated 17% to 40% of HIV infections among IDUs, their sex partners, and their children would have been prevented. Unfortunately, wide-spread N/SEPs were not implemented and the cost of the resulting HIV infections will eventually fall somewhere between $470,000 and $1,090,000. Failure to institute a national system of N/SEPs, according to these estimates, will result in 9,690 to 22,800 new cases of HIV by the year 2000.

When sterile equipment is not available and sharing is required, cleaning equipment before use can be implemented as a risk reducing activity. Cleaning can decrease, but not eliminate, the risk for those who must share equipment. It is, nevertheless, an important tactic for drug users who do not have access to sterile equipment. The recommended cleaning process follows: Fill the used syringe with full strength household bleach, shake for 30 seconds, squirt bleach out through the needle, repeat the bleaching process one more time, then rinse equipment twice with tap water. Be aware that this process takes time and may be difficult for a person in drug withdrawal.

Decreasing Risks of Perinatal Transmission

The best way to prevent HIV infection in infants is to prevent HIV infection in women (Jadeck, Hyde, & Keller, 1995; Kinsey, 1994; Lauver, Armstrong, Marks, & Schwarz, 1995). Women who are already infected with HIV should be asked about their reproductive desires. Women who choose not to have infants need to have birth control methods discussed in detail and offered abortion should they become pregnant.

HIV-infected women who choose to become pregnant or to maintain a pregnancy need to be aware of the AIDS Clinical Trials Group 076 (ACTG 076) study which showed that treating HIV-infected pregnant women and their infants with zidovudine (ZDV, AZT, Retrovir™) decreased the rate of perinatal transmission from 25.5% to 8.3% ("Antiretroviral Briefs," 1994; CDC, 1994). The study was a randomly assigned, double-blind design with placebo controls. The treatment arm provided oral zidovudine to women during the second and third trimesters of pregnancy, intravenous zidovudine during labor and delivery, and zidovudine syrup to infants during the first six weeks of life. Side effects for women taking zidovudine (headache, nausea, and fatigue) were not significantly different from women in the placebo group. The major side effect for infants was a transitory anemia that resolved upon completion of therapy (CDC, 1994). Further research is underway to determine long-term effects in these children, efficacy of focused therapy (i.e., during one specific phase of reproduction), and benefits and risks (if any) of combination antiretroviral therapy in pregnancy. The major conclusions that come from ACTG 076 are that women who are pregnant or contemplating pregnancy should be counseled about HIV infection, informed of their choices, routinely offered access to voluntary HIV antibody testing, and provided with optimal therapy as appropriate and desired (CDC, 1994).

Decreasing Risks at Work

The risk of infection from occupational exposure to HIV is small but real. Because of this, the CDC and the Occupational Safety and Health Administration (OSHA) have moved to assure that employees are protected from exposure to blood and other potentially infectious fluids. Universal Precautions (UP) are required by OSHA as the minimum protection for health care workers who have exposure risks ("Occupational Exposure," 1991). Many health care agencies use an alternative system called Body Substance Isolation (BSI), however, because it is felt to be more protective than UPs. (See Box 1.1 for an overview of the basics of BSI.) Regardless of the method used, precautions have been shown to decrease the risk of direct contact with blood and body fluids, which decreases the risk of infection from all bloodborne pathogens. Should exposure to HIV-infected fluids occur, however, treatments can be instituted. Research confirms that postexposure prophylaxis with zidovudine reduces the rate of infection from 0.3% to 0.1% (CDC, 1996) and the CDC now recommends antiretroviral post-exposure prophylaxis (PEP) based on the nature of the exposure and a broader range of antiretroviral drugs (see Table 1.2). The possibility of treatment makes immediate reporting of all blood exposures even more critical (CDC, 1996; Porche, 1997).

Table 1.1. Relative Risk of Behaviors Related to Transmission of HIV Infection

	Sexual Intercourse	Drug Use	Perinatal Transmission
SAFE BEHAVIORS (no risk of HIV transmission)	Don't have sex Limit sex to activities in which the penis, mouth, vagina, or rectum have no contact with the partner's penis, mouth, vagina, or rectum Have sex only in a mutually monogamous relationship with an uninfected partner	Don't use drugs Don't inject drugs Use only clean equipment that has not been shared with others	Prevent HIV infection in women In HIV-infected women who choose not to have children: Use birth control to prevent pregnancy Use abortion to prevent birth[1]
RISK REDUCING BEHAVIORS (decreases, but does not eliminate risk of HIV transmission)	Use barriers consistently and correctly: *Oral intercourse (male):* use nonlubricated male condoms *Oral intercourse (female):* use dental dams, plastic wrap, or latex panties *Vaginal intercourse:* use male or female condoms *Anal intercourse:* use male condoms or female condoms with inner ring removed	Clean used injection equipment before use: Rinse used needle and syringe with tap water; Fill used syringe and needle with full strength household bleach, shake for 30 seconds, squirt bleach out; repeat bleaching steps twice; Fill syringe and needle with tap water and squirt water out; repeat rinsing step twice	For HIV-infected women who choose to have children: Plan pregnancy early during infection when mother's immune status is intact Treat infected mother with appropriate anti-retroviral therapy
HIGH RISK BEHAVIORS (no protection)	Insertive sexual intercourse with an HIV-infected partner without using barriers	Share used injection equipment Have unprotected sex while under the influence of drugs (including alcohol, marijuana, and other noninjected drugs)	Pregnancy during later stages of mother's infection when immune system is more likely to be compromised

[1]Abortion is a legal option for women in the United States. It is, however, frequently not considered to be an acceptable option because of an individual's religious, cultural, ethnic, or family background. No HIV-infected woman should be forced to have an abortion. On the other hand, no HIV-infected woman should be denied an abortion if that is her choice. This difficult decision must be made by the woman using her selected resources.

Box 1.1. Body Substance Isolation (BSI)

Principles of BSI:
- Consider all moist body surfaces and substances from all patients to be potentially infectious, whether the HIV status is known or not.
  - Moist body surfaces include the mouth, vagina, and rectum as well as any open wound.
  - Moist body substances include blood, semen, vaginal secretions, sputum, saliva, urine, emesis, stool, and pericardial, synovial, amniotic, peritoneal, and cerebrospinal fluids. BSI takes into account the possibility of occult blood in fluids that do not otherwise transmit HIV or other bloodborne pathogens. BSI also protects the health care worker from organisms (such as Hepatitis A, CMV and *Salmonella*) that can be transmitted enterically.
- Avoid unprotected exposure to any moist body surface or substance.
- Use protective clothing and equipment to prevent skin and mucous membrane contamination.
  - **If hand contamination is likely, wear gloves.** For patient care, use disposable gloves that are changed frequently and discarded after completing an activity. *Gloves must be worn during all arterial and venous punctures.* Wash hands after removing gloves.
  - **If contamination of clothing is likely, wear gowns or aprons and/or shoe coverings.** Discard after use.
  - **If there is a risk that contaminated fluids will splatter into the face, use protection that covers the eyes, mouth, and nose.** A face shield or goggles and a mask can be used.
- Wash hands or other affected body parts as soon as possible after an exposure.
- Sharps must be used with extreme caution.
  - Use needle-less injection systems and automatically recapping needles as much as possible.
  - Do not recap, bend, break, or otherwise manipulate used sharps. Place used sharps into an appropriate container immediately after use.
  - If recapping is required to maintain a safe environment, use a one-handed method and dispose of the recapped needle in an appropriate container as soon as possible.
  - Sharps containers should be leak-proof, puncture-proof, and sealable. Sharps containers should be readily available in all patient care settings. Sharps containers should be sealed and sent for disposal when they are two thirds full.
- Use resuscitation equipment (masks and bags) to ventilate patients during CPR.
- Clean, disinfect, or sterilize reusable equipment according to the manufacturer's instructions between uses.

Adapted from Bradley-Springer, L., & Fendrick, R. (1994). *HIV instant instructor cards*. El Paso: Skidmore-Roth Publishing.

Table 1.2. Drug Therapy: Provisional Public Health Service recommendations for chemoprophylaxis after occupational exposure to HIV, by type of exposure and source material - 1996

(*Morbidity & Mortality Weekly Report*, volume 45, number 22, p. 471)

Type of Exposure	Source Material[1]	Antiretroviral Prophylaxis[2]	Antiretroviral Regimen[3]

Percutaneous	Blood[4]
	   Highest risk
	   Increased risk
	   No increased risk
	Fluid containing visible blood,
	   other potentially infectious fluid[5],
	   or tissue
	Other body fluid (e.g., urine)
		
		Recommend
		Recommend
		Offer
		
		Offer
		Not offer
			
			ZDV plus 3TC plus IDV
			ZDV plus 3TC +/- IDV[6]
			ZDV plus 3TC
			
			ZDV plus 3TC
			None

Mucous Membrane	Blood
	Fluid containing visible blood,
	   other potentially infectious fluid[5],
	   or tissue
	Other body fluid (e.g., urine)
		Offer
		
		Offer
		Not offer
			ZDV plus 3TC +/- IDV[6]
			
			ZDV plus 3TC
			None

Skin, increased risk[7]	Blood
	Fluid containing visible blood,
	   other potentially infectious fluid[5],
	   or tissue
	Other body fluid (e.g., urine)
		Offer
		
		Offer
		Not offer
			ZDV plus 3TC +/- IDV[6]
			
			ZDV plus 3TC
			None

[1]Any exposure to concentrated HIV (e.g., in a research laboratory or production facility) is treated as percutaneous exposure to blood with highest risk.

[2]*Recommend* - Postexposure prophylaxis (PEP) should be recommended to the exposed worker with counseling (see *MMWR*). *Offer* - PEP should be offered to the exposed worker with counseling. *Not Offer* - PEP should not be offered because these are not occupational exposures to HIV.

[3]Regimens: zidovudine (ZVD), 200 mg. PO T.I.D.; lamivudine (3TC), 150 mg. PO B.I.D.; indinavir (IDV), 800 mg. PO T.I.D. (If IDV is not available, saquinovir may be used, 600 mg PO T.I.D.) Prophylaxis is given for 4 weeks. For full prescribing information, see package inserts.

[4]*Highest Risk* - BOTH larger volume of blood (e.g., deep injury with a large diameter hollow needle previously in source-patient's vein or artery, especially involving an injection of source-patient's blood) AND blood containing a high titer of HIV (e.g., source with acute retroviral illness or end-stage AIDS; viral load measurement may be considered, but its use in relation to PEP has not been evaluated). *Increased Risk* - EITHER exposure to larger volume of blood OR blood with a higher titer of HIV. *No Increased Risk* - NEITHER exposure to larger volume of blood NOR blood with a high titer of HIV (e.g., solid suture needle injury from source-patient with asymptomatic HIV infection).

[5]Includes semen; vaginal secretions; cerebrospinal, synovial, pleural, pericardial, and amniotic fluids.

[6]Possible toxicity of additional drug may not be warranted (see *Morbidity & Mortality Weekly Report*).

[7]For skin, risk is increased for exposure involving a high titer of HIV, prolonged contact, an extensive area, or an area in which skin integrity is visibly compromised. For skin exposure without increased risk, the risk of drug toxicity outweighs the benefit of PEP.

Other Methods to Reduce Risk

It is important to encourage individuals who are at risk for HIV to be tested. Those who are found to be infected can be educated and counseled to prevent further transmissions of the virus. HIV-infected people should also be instructed to not give blood, donate organs, or donate semen for artificial insemination; to not share razors, toothbrushes, or other household items that may contain blood or other body fluids; to protect their sexual and drug using partners; and to consider reproductive counseling and/or the use of birth control measures to decrease the risk of HIV-infected children.

Spectrum of HIV Infection

HIV infection typically follows a clinical pattern of increasing immune deficiency that corresponds with decreasing CD4+ T lymphocyte counts (see Figures 1.3, 1.4, 1.5). It is important to remember, however, that HIV follows a highly individualized course. The information depicted in Figure 1.4 represents median time intervals and usual disease progression. It cannot be used to predict the progress of disease in any one HIV-infected individual.

Acute Retroviral Syndrome

Initial infection with HIV is followed within 3 weeks to 6 months by the development of detectable blood levels of HIV-specific antibodies. The development of HIV-specific antibody (or seroconversion) is frequently accompanied by a flu- or mononucleosis-like syndrome of fever, pharyngitis, headache, malaise, nausea, and a diffuse rash (Casey, 1995; Lisanti & Zwolski, 1997). These

symptoms, called acute retroviral syndrome, generally occur 1-3 weeks after initial infection and last for several weeks, although some of the symptoms may persist for several months (Staprans & Feinberg, 1997). CD4+ T lymphocyte counts will fall temporarily during this syndrome but will quickly return to baseline. This temporary decrease is a typical healthy immune response to any acute infection (Lisanti & Zwolski, 1997).

Early HIV Infection

The median time between HIV infection and a diagnosis of AIDS is 10 years. It was initially thought that this phase represented a period of biological as well as clinical latency and that viral replication was minimal. We now know, however, that HIV replication occurs at rapid and constant rates from early in the infection. During this time, CD4+ T lymphocyte counts remain normal or only slightly decreased, indicating that the body is replacing CD4+ T lymphocytes as they are destroyed by the virus. HIV-infected people remain generally healthy during early infection, but vague symptoms, including fatigue, headaches, low grade fevers, and night sweats may occur. Demyelinating peripheral neuropathies that resemble Guillain-Barré syndrome may also develop during this time (Casey et al., 1996).

Because most of the symptoms that occur during early infection are vague and non-specific for HIV, people may remain unaware that they are infected during this "asymptomatic phase." During this time, infected people continue their customary activities, which may include risky sexual and drug using behaviors. This creates a public health problem because infected people can transmit HIV to others even if they have no symptoms. This also contributes to personal health problems because unidentified infected people have no motivation to seek healthcare or make healthy lifestyle changes that could beneficially alter the quality and quantity of their lives (Flaskerud, 1995a).

Early Symptomatic Disease

Toward the end of the asymptomatic phase and before a diagnosis of AIDS, the CD4+ T lymphocyte count drops below 500-600 cells/mm³ and early symptomatic disease develops. This phase was initially called AIDS related complex (ARC), a term that is no longer used. Early symptoms can include constitutional problems such as persistent fever, recurrent drenching night sweats, chronic diarrhea, headaches, and fatigue. These may be severe enough to interrupt normal routines. Other problems that may occur at this time include localized infections, lymphadenopathy, and neurological manifestations (Casey, 1995; Staprans & Feinberg, 1997).

The most common early infection associated with HIV is oral candidiasis or thrush, a fungal infection that rarely causes problems in healthy adults. Other infections that can

occur at this time include shingles (caused by the *Varicella zoster* virus), persistent vaginal yeast infections, and outbreaks of oral or genital herpes. Oral hairy leukoplakia, an Epstein-Barr virus infection that causes painless white raised lesions on the lateral aspect of the tongue, can also occur. Oral lesions such as those seen in candida and hairy leukoplakia may provide the earliest indicators of HIV infection and are prognostic indicators of disease progression (Lisanti & Zwolski, 1997).

As the disease progresses, some infected individuals develop persistent generalized lymphadenopathy (PGL). PGL is defined as two or more enlarged lymph nodes, one centimeter or larger in size, located outside the inguinal area that persist for at least three months. PGL may continue for several years before further progression of the disease occurs (Flaskerud, 1995a).

Neurological manifestations can occur at any time during the spectrum of HIV infection, but may become more problematic during this phase. Common neurological symptoms include headache, aseptic meningitis, cranial nerve palsy, myopathy, and painful

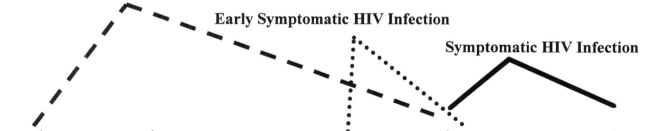

Figure 1.5. Stages in the Progression of HIV Disease.

peripheral neuropathies that may be related to HIV, other infections, neoplasms, or medication side effects (Lisanti & Zwolski, 1997). Asymptomatic neurological problems can also develop during this phase, including abnormalities in the cerebrospinal fluid (CSF), central nervous system production of HIV-specific antibody, and CSF that is HIV-culture positive (Price, 1997).

AIDS

A diagnosis of AIDS cannot be made until the HIV-infected client meets case definition criteria established by the CDC (CDC, 1992). These criteria, listed in Box 1.2, are more likely to occur when the immune system becomes severely compromised. As the disease progresses, the CD4+ T lymphocyte count decreases and the ratio of CD4 to CD8 cells (helper to suppressor cells) gradually reverses, resulting in more suppressor than helper cells. There is an increase in the amount of HIV that can be detected in the blood and there may be decreases in the absolute number of lymphocytes as well as the percent of lymphocytes. Skin test reactivity decreases or disappears and immunoglobulin levels increase (Grady & Vogel, 1993).

The median time for survival after a diagnosis of AIDS is two years but this varies greatly. Some people with AIDS live for six or more years while others survive for only a few months. There is also a wide variation in morbidity. Some people with AIDS are severely ill and are considered terminal while others are able to continue their routines making modifications to compensate for fatigue, pain, bouts of diarrhea, or other manageable problems (Staprans & Feinberg, 1997). Advances in the treatment and diagnosis of HIV infection, opportunistic diseases, and constitutional symptoms have increased survival times, resulting in the

recent decreases in death rates attributed to AIDS in the United States (CDC, 1998). Despite advances, however, HIV disease remains an incurable process that complicates all aspects of life for HIV-infected people.

Medical Management of HIV Infection

Therapeutic management of HIV-infected patients has become more complex since 1994 because of advances in laboratory analysis of health status and the development of new antiretroviral drug therapies. Current therapy focuses on monitoring HIV disease progression and immune function, initiating and monitoring antiretroviral therapy (ART), preventing the development of opportunistic diseases, detecting and treating opportunistic diseases, managing symptoms, and preventing complications of treatment. Continuing assessment and clinician-patient interactions are required to accomplish these objectives (Barlett, 1996; Masci, 1996). See Table 1.3 for a summary of assessment parameters that need to be accomplished during course of HIV disease.

The initial visit provides an opportunity to gather baseline data and to establish rapport. A complete history and physical exam, including an immunization history and psychosocial and dietary evaluations should be conducted. Findings from the history, assessment, and laboratory tests will help to determine the patient's needs. This is a good time to initiate patient education related to the spectrum of HIV disease, treatments, preventing transmission to others, improving immune health, and family planning. Patient input should be used to develop a plan of care and necessary referrals can be made.

It is important to remember that a newly diagnosed client may be in a state of shock or denial (Masci, 1996) and unable to retain or synthesize information (Flaskerud, 1995b). Be prepared to repeat and clarify information over the course of several months.

Drug Therapy for HIV Infection

The goals of pharmacologic therapy in HIV infection are to: 1) decrease HIV RNA levels to less than 5000 copies/mm^3 (undetectable HIV RNA levels are possible and preferred); 2) maintain or raise CD4$^+$ T lymphocyte counts to greater than 500 cells/mm^3 (a range of 800-1200 cells/mm^3 is preferred); and 3) delay the development of HIV-related symptoms including a wide range of opportunistic diseases. A variety of pharmacologic therapies is now available to help patients meet these goals. Because of the rapidity with which new therapies are evolving, there has been considerable confusion about how and when to use antiretroviral therapy. The National Institutes of Health (NIH, 1997) has published a report on the principles of therapy, as summarized in Box 1.3. Guidelines on the use of antiretroviral agents have also been published (Panel on Clinical Practices, 1997). Recommendations for the initiation of therapy in the chronically infected patient are summarized in Table 1.4.

Drugs in three different pharmacologic groups have now been approved to treat HIV infection. Research is progressing rapidly to develop new groups of drugs, new drugs in the established categories, and new systems for drug delivery to target sites (Martin, 1996). At present, no drug or combination of drugs can cure HIV, but new therapies can decrease viral replication (as evidenced by lowered viral loads) and delay progression of disease in many

patients. The major advantage of having antiretroviral drugs from different drug groups is that combination therapy, which increases efficacy and decreases the likelihood of drug resistance, is now available (Williams, 1997). An additional advantage is that alternatives now exist for those patients who fail to respond to a specific drug regimen (Panel on Clinical Practices, 1997; Ungvarski, 1997).

The three currently approved groups of drugs include two that inhibit the ability of HIV to make a DNA copy early in replication and one that inhibits the ability of the virus to produce viable virions in the late stages of replication (see Table 1.5). Nucleoside reverse transcriptase inhibitors (NRTIs) and non-nucleoside reverse transcriptase inhibitors (NNRTIs) both work by inhibiting the activity of the enzyme reverse transcriptase, while protease inhibitors (PIs) work by interfering with the work of the protease enzyme (Williams, 1997). A major problem with stavudine (an NRTI) and the PIs is that resistance develops rapidly when they are used alone. For that reason, these drugs must always be used in combination with other drugs and must be taken on a strictly adhered-to schedule (Wilson, 1997). PIs and NNRTIs also have a number of dangerous and potentially lethal interactions with commonly used drugs (Jones & Gelone, 1997; Lisanti & Zwolski, 1997; Panel on Clinical Practices, 1997).

Because treatment with new drug combinations has resulted in dramatic improvements in many HIV-infected clients, current therapeutic recommendations are for combination antiretroviral therapy with at least three drugs, preferably two NRTIs and one PI. Monotherapy is generally not recommended unless extenuating circumstances are documented. While the research on these treatment protocols is generally very good, with

Box 1.2. Diagnostic criteria for AIDS

AIDS is diagnosed when an individual with HIV develops at least one of these additional conditions:

- The CD4$^+$ T lymphocyte count drops below 200/mm^3.

- The development of one of the following opportunistic infections (OIs):

  > Fungal: *Pneumocystis carinii* pneumonia (PCP); candidiasis of bronchi, trachea, lungs or esophagus; disseminated or extrapulmonary coccidioidomycosis, disseminated or extrapulmonary histoplasmosis; *Cryptococcus neoformans* meningitis or extrapulmonary cryptococcosis
  > Viral: cytomegalovirus (CMV) disease other than liver, spleen or nodes; CMV retinitis (with loss of vision); herpes simplex with chronic ulcer(s) or bronchitis, pneumonitis or esophagitis; progressive multifocal leukoencephalopathy (PML)
  > Protozoal: toxoplasmosis of the brain, chronic intestinal isosporiasis; chronic intestinal cryptosporidiosis
  > Bacterial: *Mycobacterium tuberculosis* (any site); any disseminated or extrapulmonary *Mycobacterium*, including *M. avium* complex or *M. kansasii;* recurrent pneumonia; recurrent *Salmonella* septicemia, Nocardiosis

- The development of one of the following opportunistic cancers: invasive cervical cancer, Kaposi's sarcoma (KS), Burkitt's Lymphoma, immunoblastic lymphoma, or primary lymphoma of the brain

- Wasting syndrome, defined as a loss of 10% or more of ideal body mass

- Dementia: AIDS dementia complex (ADC) causes neurocognitive deficits and behavioral symptoms that are not related to other causes

Modified from: Centers for Disease Control and Prevention (CDC). (1992, December 18). Recommendations and Reports: 1993 revised classification system for HIV infection and expanded surveillance case definition for AIDS among adolescents and adults. *Morbidity and Mortality Weekly Report, 41* (RR-17), 1-17.

Table 1.3. Baseline and Follow-Up Assessment Parameters in HIV Infection

PARAMETERS	Initial Visit	CD4 >500	CD4 <500	CD4 <200	CD4 <100
Office visit	follow-up in 2 weeks	q 3-6 mos	q 2-3 mos	q 1-2 mos	PRN
CBC with differential & platelet count	✓	q 3-6 mos	q 2-3 mos	q 1-2 mos	PRN
Chemistry panel (SMA 12, 14, or 20)	✓	q 3-6 mos	q 2-3 mos	q 1-2 mos	PRN
Amylase		monthly if patient is on didanosine			
RPR or VDRL	✓	annually as long as patient is sexually active			
CD4+ T lymphocyte count	✓	q 3-6 mos	q 1-3 mos	q 1-3 mos	PRN
Viral load assessment (bDNA or PCR)[1]	✓	as indicated to initiate and monitor therapy			
Hepatitis B serology	✓				
Toxoplasma & CMV serologies (IgG)	✓			✓	
AFB, blood culture	✓			✓	✓
Chest X-ray	✓			✓	PRN
PPD skin test by Mantoux method	✓	if negative at baseline, repeat annually; consider q 6 month testing in high prevalence areas			
Family planning/contraception	discuss	discuss with each visit as needed			
Pelvic with Pap/Colposcopy	✓	annual	q 6 mos	q 6 mos/PRN	q 6 mos/PRN
Mammogram	✓	annually for rest of life			
Eye exam by ophthalmologic consult	✓	annual	annual	q 6 mos	q 4-6 mos
Dental exam/prophylaxis	oral exam at each visit; dental care q 3-6 months for cleaning and as needed				

Adapted from Bradley-Springer LA, Fendrick R: *HIV instant instructor cards.* El Paso, 1994, Skidmore-Roth Publishing.

[1] Viral loads should be assessed immediately prior to and 4 weeks after initiation or change in antiretroviral therapy. A greater than 10 fold (1 log) decrease in viral load will indicate successful therapy. With optimal therapy, viral load should be undetectable at 6 months (Panel on Clinical Practices, 1997).

Box 1.3. Summary of the Principles of Therapy of HIV Infection

1. Ongoing HIV replication leads to immune system damage and progression to AIDS. HIV infection is always harmful, and true long-term survival free of clinically significant immune dysfunction is unusual.
2. Plasma HIV RNA levels indicate the magnitude of HIV replication and its associated rate of CD4$^+$ T-cell destruction, while CD4$^+$ T-cell counts indicate the extent of HIV-induced immune damage already suffered. Regular, periodic measurement of plasma HIV RNA levels and CD4$^+$ T-cell counts is necessary to determine the risk of disease progression in an HIV-infected individual and to determine when to initiate or modify antiretroviral treatment regimens.
3. As rates of disease progression differ among individuals, treatment decisions should be individualized by level of risk indicated by plasma HIV RNA levels and CD4$^+$ T-cell counts.
4. The use of potent combination antiretroviral therapy to suppress HIV replication to below the levels of detection of sensitive plasma HIV RNA assays limits the potential for selection of antiretroviral-resistant HIV variants, the major factor limiting the ability of antiretroviral drugs to inhibit virus replication and delay disease progression. Therefore, maximum achievable suppression of HIV replication should be the goal of therapy.
5. The most effective means to accomplish durable suppression of HIV replication is the simultaneous initiation of combinations of effective anti-HIV drugs with which the patient has not been previously treated and that are not cross-resistant with antiretroviral agents with which the patient has been previously treated.
6. Each of the antiretroviral drugs used in combination therapy regimens should always be used according to optimum schedules and dosages.
7. The available effective antiretroviral drugs are limited in number and mechanism of action and cross-resistance between specific drugs has been documented. Therefore, any change in antiretroviral therapy increases future therapeutic constraints.
8. Women should receive optimal antiretroviral therapy regardless of pregnancy status.
9. The same principles of antiretroviral therapy apply to both HIV-infected children and adults, although the treatment of HIV-infected children involves unique pharmacologic, virologic, and immunologic considerations.
10. Persons with acute primary HIV infections should be treated with combination antiretroviral therapy to suppress virus replication to levels below the limit of detection of sensitive plasma HIV RNA assays.
11. HIV-infected persons, even those with viral loads below detectable limits, should be considered infectious and should be counseled to avoid sexual and drug-use behaviors that are associated with transmission or acquisition of HIV and other infectious pathogens.

Revised from the *Report of the NIH Panel to Define Principles of Therapy of HIV Infection*, National Institutes of Health (NIH, 1997).

Table 1.4. Drug Therapy: Indications for the Initiation of Antiretroviral Therapy in the Chronically HIV-Infected Patient[1]

Clinical Category	CD4+ T lymphocyte Count & HIV RNA Level	Recommendation
Symptomatic (AIDS diagnosis, thrush, or unexplained fever)	Any value	Treat.
Asymptomatic	CD4+ T lymphocytes <500/mm³ **or** HIV RNA >10,000 (dDNA) or >20,000 (RT-PCR)	Treatment should be offered. Strength of recommendation is based on prognosis for disease-free survival as demonstrated in research and willingness of the patient to accept and comply with therapy.[2]
Asymptomatic	CD4+ T lymphocytes >500/uL **and** HIV RNA <10,000 (bDNA) or <20,000 (RT-PCR)	Some experts would delay therapy and observe; however, some experts would treat.

[1]Revised from the Guidelines for the Use of Antiretroviral Agents in HIV-Infected Adults and Adolescents (Panel of Clinical Practice, 1997).

[2]Some experts would observe patients with CD4+ T lymphocyte counts between 350-500/mm³ and HIV RNA levels <10,000 (bDNA) or <20,000 (RT-PCR).

Table 1.5. Drug Therapy: Antiretroviral Agents Used in HIV Infection
(Bartlett, 1998; Jones & Gelone, 1997; Panel on Clinical Practice, 1997; Williams, 1997.)

DRUG/ADMINISTRATION	ADVERSE EFFECTS	COMMENTS/DRUG INTERACTIONS
Nucleoside Reverse Transcriptase Inhibitors (NRTIs):		
Zidovudine (AZT, ZDV, Retrovir™) - 200 mg po t.i.d. or 300 mg po b.i.d. Take with meals to decrease nausea and vomiting.	fatigue, malaise, headache, nausea, vomiting, insomnia, malaise, myalgia; bone marrow suppression: anemia, neutropenia; nail pigmentation, myopathy	Although blood dyscrasias are not common at current dosages, anemia can be treated with transfusions or erythropoietin (EPO); granulocytopenia can be treated with granulocyte colony-stimulating factor (G-CSF). Use with caution with other bone marrow suppressing drugs. Do not use in combination with stavudine.
Didanosine (ddI, Videx™) - dose by weight: > 60 kg - 200 mg po b.i.d.; < 60 kg - 125 mg po b.i.d. Dose must be provided in 2 tablets to assure adequate buffer for absorption. Tablets must be chewed or dissolved to release buffer. Take 1/2 hour before or 1-2 hours after eating.	dry mouth, altered taste, diarrhea, pancreatitis, painful peripheral neuropathy (dose related and reversible), abdominal pain, rash, oral ulcers	Avoid alcohol which may exacerbate pancreatitis. Avoid H_2 antagonists, antacids, and omeprazole. Not recommended for use with Zalcitabine. Drugs that require gastric acidity for absorption should be taken 2 hours before or after ddI; these include protease inhibitors, indinavir, dapsone, quinolones.
Zalcitabine (ddC, HIVID™) - 0.75 mg po t.i.d.	painful peripheral neuropathy, aphthous ulcers, pancreatitis, rash, fever, hepatitis	Overlapping toxicity with ddI, d4T, and other drugs causing peripheral neuropathy. Avoid alcohol which may exacerbate pancreatitis.
Stavudine (d4T, Zerit™) - dose by weight: > 60 kg - 40 mg po b.i.d.; < 60 kg - 30 mg po b.i.d.	painful peripheral neuropathy (dose related and reversible), pancreatitis, elevated liver enzymes, nausea, diarrhea	Not recommended for use with zidovudine. Overlapping toxicity with ddI, ddC, and other drugs causing peripheral neuropathy. Avoid alcohol which may exacerbate pancreatitis.
Lamivudine (3TC, Epivir™) - 150 mg po b.i.d.; adults <50 Kg - 2 mg/kg po b.i.d.	minimal toxicity: mild rash, headache, diarrhea, hair loss, insomnia, nausea	High level resistance develops rapidly, use only in combination regimens. Not recommended for use with zalcitabine.
Zidovudine & lamivudine (Combivir™) - 1 tab 300 mg ZDV & 150 mg 3TC) po b.i.d.	potential side effects to both drugs (see above)	Decreases number of pills taken each day; simplifies drug-taking regimens. Not recommended for use with stavudine.
Abacavir (Ziagen) - 300 mg po b.i.d.	hypersensitivity reaction, fever, nausea, vomiting, malaise, rash	If hypersensitivity reaction occurs, DO NOT re-challenge (may be life-threatening).
Adefovir dipivoxil (Preveon™) - 60 mg or 120 mg po qd (FDA approval pending)	Fanconi syndrome and renal failure common with prolonged use or high dose (120 mg/d)	Monitor renal function, serum phosphate, and urinalysis for glycosuria and proteinuria.

DRUG/ADMINISTRATION	ADVERSE EFFECTS	COMMENTS/DRUG INTERACTIONS
Non-Nucleoside Reverse Transcriptase Inhibitors (NNRTIs): As a group, NNRTIs have multiple drug interactions with some analgesics, cardiac drugs, antimicrobial agents, nonsedating antihistamines, antidepressants, psychotropics, vasoconstrictors, and oral contraceptives as well as with other antiretroviral agents. Care should be taken to consult with a pharmacist or a current text when these drugs are prescribed.		
Nevirapine (Viramune™) - lead-in dose - 200 mg po qd x 14 days, followed by 200 mg po b.i.d.	rash, fever, nausea, headache, increased liver enzymes, thrombocytopenia, Stevens-Johnson syndrome, myalgia	Be aware of drug interactions.
Delavirdine (Rescriptor™) - 400 mg po t.i.d. Mix tablets in 3 or more ounces of water to produce a slurry.	rash, fever, pruritis, headache, fatigue, nausea, vomiting, diarrhea, elevated liver enzymes	Be aware of drug interactions. Separate from doses of antacids and didanosine by one or more hours.
Efavirenz (Sustiva™) - 600 mg po qd.	dizziness, "disconnected feeling," somnolence, impaired concentration, insomnia, impaired dreaming, rash usually resolved in 2-4 weeks	Recommend qd dose to be taken at bed time for better tolerance of side effects; limited data on drug interactions, but there are reduced levels of clarithromycin and indinavir with concurrent use and increased levels of nelfinavir with concurrent use.
Protease Inhibitors (PIs): Resistance develops rapidly; recommended for use in combination therapy only; no skipped doses; no drug holidays. As a group, PIs have multiple drug interactions with some analgesics, cardiac drugs, anti-microbial agents, nonsedating antihistamines, antidepressants, psychotropics, vaso-constrictors, and oral contraceptives as well as with other antiretroviral agents. Care should be taken to consult with a pharmacist or a current text when these drugs are prescribed.		
Saquinovir (Fortovase™) - 1200 mg po t.i.d. Take with meals or within 2 hours of eating a full meal (including proteins, fats, and carbohydrates).	diarrhea, abdominal pain, nausea, heartburn, headache, elevated transaminase enzymes	Be aware of drug interactions. Grapefruit juice increases bioavailability.
Indinavir (IDV, Crixivan™) - 800 mg po q8h.	kidney stones (flank pain with or without hematuria), nausea, vomiting, diarrhea, headache, fatigue, insomnia, metallic taste, asymptomatic hyperbilirubinemia	Be aware of drug interactions. Assure adequate hydration during therapy; patient should drink 2-4 liters of fluid a day. Administer on an empty stomach or with a light, nonfat meal. Do not take in conjunction with grapefruit juice which decreases bioavailability.
Ritonivir (Norvir™) - 600 mg po q12h. Preferable to give with food, but not required; dose escalation may be required.	nausea, diarrhea, vomiting, anorexia, abdominal pain, taste perversion, circumoral and peripheral paresthesias, elevations in triglycerides, transaminase levels, CPK, and uric acid	Be aware of drug interactions which are more numerous with this drug. Keep capsules refrigerated. (Single dose may be kept at room temperature for up to 12 hours.) Taking with chocolate milk decreases bitter aftertaste.
Nelfinavir (Viracept™) - 750 mg po q8h. Take with meal or light snack.	diarrhea, nausea, back pain, fever, headache, malaise, anorexia, anemia	Be aware of drug interactions.

viral loads being reduced by 90% - 99% (1-3 log decreases in viral loads) in many cases (Panel on Clinical Practices, 1997), there are some problems. At least 20%, and maybe as many as 50%, of patients with HIV will not experience a dramatic response to the drugs, causing feelings of guilt, despair, and futility. In addition, many patients will not be able to use combination therapies because of the expense, side effects, or inability to follow the stringent schedules and dietary prescriptions required with these therapies. Expense is a major concern for many, although economic analysis suggests that combination antiretroviral therapy is more cost effective than the price of advancing disease (Moore & Bartlett, 1996). The outlook is improving, but there is, as yet, no magic bullet (Bradley-Springer, 1997b).

Because resistance to antiretroviral drugs is a major problem in treating HIV infection, nurses must be prepared to provide information and constant encouragement to clients who are using combination therapies. Clients should be taught the following key points to decrease the risk of developing resistance:

- Clients should expect to be taking three different kinds of antiretroviral drugs at a time. Other options (i.e., monotherapy, or combinations of 2 or 4 drugs) may need to be used, but all therapies should be discussed thoroughly with the physician or nurse practitioner prior to implementation.
- Be sure that clients know what drugs they are taking and how to take them (some have to be taken with food, some must be taken on an empty stomach, some cannot be taken together). Ask for feedback from the client; provide clearly written instructions; and give the client a phone number to call if questions arise.

- The full doses of all prescribed drugs must be taken and they must be taken on schedule. Teach clients to report problems and side effects to a physician or nurse practitioner; adjustments can only be made if the prescribing practitioner is aware of problems.
- Many antiretroviral drugs interact with other drugs, including a number of common medications that can be obtained without a prescription. Encourage clients to disclose all medications to the physician or nurse practitioner. Before using any new medication, the client should ask about possible interactions.

Drug Therapy for Opportunistic Diseases

Management of HIV is complicated by the many opportunistic diseases that can develop as the immune system deteriorates. While new antiretroviral therapies help to decrease the occurrence of these diseases, once contracted, they can be deadly. Although it is usually not possible to eradicate opportunistic diseases, treatments that can prevent and control them are available, and advances in the diagnosis and treatment of opportunistic diseases have contributed significantly to increased life expectancy. Table 1.6 lists treatments for common opportunistic diseases in HIV-infected individuals. Because there are no cures for these diseases, suppressive therapy, when instituted, must continue for life. Stopping therapy can result in the reappearance of the condition (CDC, 1997).

Obviously, a preferred approach to opportunistic diseases would be to prevent their occurrences in the first place. A number of opportunistic diseases associated with HIV can be delayed or prevented through the use

Table 1.6. Drug Therapy: Common Opportunistic Diseases Associated with AIDS
(Bartlett, 1996; CDC, 1997)

Organism/Disease	Clinical Manifestations	Diagnostic Tests	Treatment
RESPIRATORY SYSTEM			
Pneumocystis carinii pneumonia (PCP)	nonproductive cough, hypoxemia, progressive short-ness of breath, fever, night sweats, fatigue	CXR, induced sputum for culture, bron-choalveolar lavage	trimethoprim-sulfamethoxazole (TMP-SMX), pentamidine, dapsone + trimethoprim, clin-damycin + primaquine, atovaquone, trime-trexate + folinic acid +/– dapsone, steroids
Histoplasma capsulatum	Pneumonia, fever, cough, weight loss; disseminated disease	Sputum culture, serum or urine antigen assay	amphotericin B, itroconazole, fluconazole
Mycobacterium tuberculosis	Productive cough, fever, night sweats, weight loss	CXR, sputum for AFB stain & culture	isoniazid, ethambutol, rifampin, pyrazinamide, streptomycin
Coccidioides immitis	Fever, weight loss, cough	Sputum culture, serology	amphotericin B, fluconazole, itroconazole, ketoconazole
Kaposi's sarcoma (KS)	Dyspnea, respiratory failure	CXR, biopsy	chemotherapy, alpha-interferon, radiation
INTEGUMENTARY SYSTEM			
Herpes simplex, type 1 (HSV1) & type 2 (HSV2)	Orolabial mucocutaneous ulcerative lesions; genital & perianal mucocutaneous ulcerative lesions	Viral culture	acyclovir, foscarnet
Varicella zoster virus (VZV)	Shingles: erythematous maculopapular rash along dermatomal planes, pain, pruritis	Viral culture	acyclovir, foscarnet
Kaposi's sarcoma (KS)	Firm, flat, raised or nodular, hyperpigmented, multicentric lesions	Biopsy of lesions	chemotherapy, alpha-interferon, radiation
Bacillary angiomatosis	Erythematous vascular papules, subcutaneous nodules	Biopsy of lesions	Erythromycin, doxycycline
EYE			
Cytomegalovirus (CMV)	Lesions on the retina, blurred vision, loss of vision	Ophthalmoscopic exam	ganciclovir, foscarnet, cidofovir + probenecid
Herpes virus, 1 (HSV1)	Blurred vision, corneal lesions, acute retinal necrosis	Ophthalmoscopic exam	acyclovir, foscarnet
Varicella zoster virus (VZV)	Ocular lesions, acute retinal necrosis	Ophthalmoscopic exam	acyclovir, foscarnet

Organism/Disease	Clinical Manifestations	Diagnostic Tests	Treatment
GASTROINTESTINAL SYSTEM			
Cryptosporidium muris	Watery diarrhea, abdominal pain, weight loss, nausea	Stool exam, small bowel or colon biopsy	antidiarrheals, paromomycin, azithromycin, atovaquone, octreotide
Cytomegalovirus (CMV)	Stomatitis, esophagitis, gastritis, colitis, bloody diarrhea, pain, weight loss	Endoscopy, culture, biopsy, r/o other causes	ganciclovir, foscarnet
Herpes simplex, 1 (HSV1)	Vesicular eruptions on tongue, buccal, pharyngeal, or perioral esophageal mucosa	Viral culture	acyclovir, foscarnet
Candida albicans	Whitish-yellow patches in mouth, esophagus, GI tract	Microscopic exam of lesion scraping, culture	nystatin, clotrimazole, ketoconazole, fluconazole, itroconazole, Amphotericin B
Mycobacterium avium complex (MAC)	Watery diarrhea, weight loss	Small bowel biopsy with AFB stain & culture	rifabutin, clarithromycin, rifampin, ciprofloxacin, clofamizine, amikacin, ethambutol, azithromycin
Isospora belli	Diarrhea, weight loss, nausea, abdominal pain	Stool exam, small-bowel or colon biopsy	TMP-SMX, pyrimethamine + folinic acid
Salmonella	Gastroenteritis, fever, diarrhea	Blood & stool culture	ampicillin, amoxicillin, ciprofloxacin, TMP-SMX
Kaposi's sarcoma (KS)	Diarrhea, hyperpigmented lesions of mouth & GI tract	GI series, biopsy	chemotherapy, alpha-interferon, radiation
Non-Hodgkin's lymphoma	Abdominal pain, fever, night sweats, weight loss	Lymph node biopsy	chemotherapy
NEUROLOGICAL SYSTEM			
Toxoplasma gondii	Cognitive dysfunction, motor impairment, fever, altered mental status, headache, seizures	MRI, CT scan, serology, brain biopsy	pyrimethamine + folic acid, sulfadiazine, clindamycin, azithromycin, clarithromycin
JC papovavirus	Progressive multifocal leukoencephalopathy (PML), mental & motor declines	MRI, CT scan, brain biopsy	effective antiretroviral therapy may help
Cryptococcal meningitis	Cognitive impairment, motor dysfunction, fever, seizures, headache	CT scan, antigen test, CSF analysis	amphotericin B, flucytosine, fluconazole, itroconazole
CNS lymphomas	Cognitive dysfunction, motor impairment, aphasia, seizures, personality changes, headache	MRI, CT scan	radiation, steroids
AIDS-dementia complex	Insidious onset of progressive dementia	CT scan	effective antiretroviral therapy may help

of adequate antiretroviral management and disease-specific prophylactic interventions. Prophylaxis has contributed significantly to the decreased morbidity and mortality associated with HIV infection over the past several years and is recommended according to established criteria (see Table 1.7) (Bartlett, 1996; CDC, 1997).

Table 1.7. Drug Therapy: Prophylactic Interventions for Patients with HIV Infection
(Bartlett, 1996; CDC, 1997b; Masci, 1996)

Problem	Prophylactic Interventions	Comments
Hepatitis B virus (HBV)	hepatitis B vaccine series; screen and vaccinate those who show no evidence of previous HBV infection	Provide as soon as possible during course of infection. Encourage vaccine in injecting drug users, sexually active MSM, and sex partners or household contacts of HBV-infected individuals.
Influenza virus	whole or split virus vaccine	Provide annually, before influenza virus season.
Mycobacterium avium complex (MAC)	clarithromycin or azithromycin (preferred); rifabutin	Initiate when CD4+ T lymphocytes go below 50/mm³. Rule out disseminated disease or tuberculosis. Rifabutin has caused dose-related uveitis (above 600 mg/day) that is reversible with drug withdrawal or dose reduction.
Mycobacterium tuberculosis	treat if PPD is >5 mm reactive, after high-risk exposure, or if prior positive PPD without treatment; INH + pyridoxine for 12 months; consider directly observed therapy.	Rule out active disease, extrapulmonary disease, or drug resistant strain, all of which require multi-drug therapy. Remember that a negative PPD in the presence of HIV does not exclude a diagnosis of TB. Provide ongoing assessment and intervention.
Pneumococcal pneumonia	pneumococcal vaccine with 23-valent vaccine; use of prophylaxis for PCP and MAC also decreases risk	Provide as soon as possible during course of infection: antibody response is optimal when CD4+ T lymphocytes are >350/mm³.
Pneumocystis carinii pneumonia (PCP)	TMP-SMX (preferred) or dapsone, dapsone with pyrimethamine + folic acid, or aerosolized pentamidine	Initiate when CD4+ T lymphocytes go below 200/mm³. Offer to any patient with a history of PCP, fever of undetermined origin for 2 or more weeks, or oropharyngeal candidiasis regardless of CD4+ T lymphocyte count. Oral drugs which provide systemic effect are preferred. Side effects of TMP-SMX and dapsone, especially rash and fever, are common and may limit use.
Toxoplasmosis	TMP-SMX or dapsone with pyrimethamine + folic acid	Initiate with positive toxoplasmosis IgG titer when CD4+ T lymphocytes go below 100/mm³.
Varicella zoster virus (VZV)	varicella zoster immune globulin (VZIG) administered within 96 hours after an exposure	Only after significant exposure to chicken pox or shingles for patients with no history of disease or negative on a VZV antibody test.

Chapter II

Nursing Management of HIV Infection

HIV infection provides unlimited opportunities for nurse caring in all health care settings including acute, chronic, long term, institutional, community, home, and mental health. HIV requires that nurses provide care as practitioners, advocates, educators, collaborators, and researchers at all levels of disease prevention, health promotion, and caring intervention. Nurse caring in HIV infection is based, as is all nurse caring, on positive regard, client assessment, problem identification, and cooperatively planned interventions. This book is based on fundamental concepts that are important to nursing in general and to nursing in the HIV epidemic in particular, including disease prevention and health promotion, behavior change and adherence issues, chronicity, and holistic nursing care, all of which interact to form a focused approach to individualized client care.

Disease Prevention and Health Promotion

Disease prevention and health promotion are effective health care strategies for most health care problems including HIV infection. This book is structured around the concept of nursing care at various levels of prevention. The focus of care at the primary prevention level is to prevent new cases of HIV infection and decrease risks of transmission. Major interventions at this level include education and skill development for behavior change. Nursing care at the secondary prevention level focuses on HIV-infected clients. The goal at this level is to slow or prevent disease progression through activities that enhance wellness and immune function. At the tertiary prevention level the focus shifts to preventing morbidity and disability while delaying death. Nursing

care in the terminal phase focuses on enhancing comfort and dignity during the dying process.

The book is divided into sections that focus on each of these levels: primary prevention, secondary prevention, tertiary prevention, and, finally, terminal disease. Nursing goals and overview materials are provided at the beginning of each section, followed by assessment information, nursing diagnoses, and interventions appropriate to each level. It is important to point out that all categorization systems are artificial and to remember that there is considerable overlap of care needs in HIV disease. The conceptual structure of this book, therefore, merely provides a simplified way of looking at issues that the author acknowledges to be extremely complex.

Behavior Change and Adherence Issues

Nurses have been dealing with the issue of client adherence (formerly referred to as compliance) for centuries. Anytime clients are asked to change and/or maintain new behaviors to treat an existing condition or to prevent a threatened one, there is a good chance that they will not comply "consistently and correctly" to the prescribed activities. In reality, adherence is merely a part of the process of behavior change, a difficult and time consuming endeavor. These issues are important to nurses because nurses have major roles to play in helping clients change and maintain behaviors to improve health outcomes. The HIV epidemic has pointed out a number of areas in which behavior change and adherence are important processes such as developing and using safer sex methods, cleaning injection equipment, instituting diet and exercise programs, and taking multidrug therapy on time and as ordered so as to prevent the development of drug resistance, to name a few. Unfortunately, developing and maintaining new behaviors is a difficult and cumbersome process, so it will help the nurse to work from the structure of a behavior change model.

One functional model in HIV infection is the Transtheoretical Model, which incorporates principles of harm reduction, self-esteem enhancement, client autonomy, decision making, and focused interventions. The Transtheoretical Model provides a basis for understanding behavior change and for developing interventions to help clients move toward change. The central premise of the Transtheoretical Model, also known as the Stages of Change Theory, is that people progress through a series of stages when they attempt to change behaviors. Prochaska, Redding, Harlow, Rossi, and Velicer (1994) identified the following five stages of change: precontemplation, contemplation, preparation, action, and maintenance. Knowing that stages exist provides an interesting piece of information. The key to the utility of this model, however, lies in identifying the client's current stage and using this information to develop appropriate interventions. Table 2.1 provides an overview of the Transtheoretical Model including stage appropriate interventions that can be incorporated into helping clients decrease their risks for HIV infection (Bradley-Springer, 1996).

Adherence to prescribed therapies has been an issue for most of the HIV epidemic, starting with the earliest studies on zidovudine and continuing with discoveries related to pneumocystis prophylaxis. What is now driving the literature about treatment adherence in the care of people infected with HIV is new multidrug antiretroviral therapy (ART) that has the potential to significantly decrease viral loads, increase CD4+ T lymphocytes, and improve the quality and quantity of life for infected individuals. Unfortunately, treatment protocols that are not followed judiciously have the potential result of partial viral inhibition leading to the development of drug-resistant virus, cross resistance to related drugs, and, of equal concern, transmission of drug-resistance viruses to others. It has become clear in a very short period of time that adherence is a critical issue (Britten, 1994; Crespo-Fiero, 1997; Klaus & Grodesky, 1997; Olfson, Hansell, & Boyer, 1997).

What we know about adherence from clients with other conditions (especially tuberculosis, psychiatric disorders, and aging-related problems) is that this is not a simple issue. We know that many factors can decrease rates of adherence, that those factors occur in unique combinations for each individual client, and that most HIV-infected clients will have one or more of these barriers. Some of these barriers are related to personal attributes such as a history of drug or alcohol dependence; denial of the severity of the illness; tentative or conditional acceptance of the behavior change; denial of the need for change; impaired physical, mental, or emotional functioning; a generally negative orientation to health care (including distrust, dislike, suspicion, lack of confidence, fear); feelings of powerlessness; and language barriers including the inability to understand specific languages or medical jargon in spoken or written forms. Environmental factors that can affect behavior change and maintenance include cultural values and beliefs that differ from those of the health care provider; economic constraints (including the inability to afford treatments and follow-up care, homelessness, unemployment); social barriers (including safety issues related to confidentiality, embarrassment, disease-related stigma); barriers to health care (including inconvenient, inaccessible, or inflexible clinical settings, paternalistic

Table 2.1. Transtheoretical Model of Change

Stage: Client's Perspective	Relapse	Interventions
Precontemplation: unaware of or unwilling to consider the problem; defensive about the change issue, resistant to information about the behavior, and reluctant to initiate a behavior change program; not considering change within the next 6 months	Not a problem.	Raise awareness of the issue through community-appropriate public education and media programs. Provide information and feedback to increase individual awareness of physical, social, economic, and psychological problems related to the commission or omission of specific behaviors. Discuss the positive aspects of change. Do not spend time discussing details of specific change tactics or programs; you're wasting your time if it is clear that the client is not ready to think about changing.
Contemplation: ambivalent; frequently responds with "Yes, but . . ."; may see reasons to change as well as reasons to remain the same; indecisive and lacks commitment, but aware that a problem exists and more open to information; intends to change behavior within next 6 months		Tip the balance in favor of change. It is important to see this stage as the time when the client will develop a commitment to change. It is still too early to focus on strategies at this point - focus should be on analyzing risks and rewards of the behavior and on providing information. Clarify goals and discuss incentives to change. It is now time to emphasize negative aspects of not changing. This is when a discussion of the risk for HIV infection or the problems of further immune suppression for already infected clients is appropriate.
Preparation: expresses determination to do something to initiate change; some experimentation with new behaviors may already be occurring; seriously planning change within next 30 days, but has not reached specific criterion	Relapse is a real possibility. Clients may get "stuck" in relapse if they resort to self-blame or self-incrimination. Help the client renew the change process at an earlier stage without getting demoralized. Explain that relapse is not unusual and may occur many times before behavior change is permanent.	Now is the time to get down to details. Help the client find change strategies that are acceptable, appropriate, and effective. Encourage the client to experiment with a strategy: "Try it next time, see how you like it," or "Find out how your family/partner/friends react when you do it." Be available to the client to discuss any issues related to making a concerted effort to move into the action stage. Help client establish specific criterion such as never sharing injection equipment, eating three snacks a day, or exercising three times a week.
Action: engages in action to create desired change; behavior modified to specific criterion for 6 months		Support change efforts. This is not an easy process. Clients will need continuing encouragement, help with problem solving, and a place to simply vent frustrations.
Maintenance: challenged to continue change; continues behavior change for more than 6 months		Help client maintain change and prevent relapse. Identify and use strategies to prevent relapse. Problem solving and unconditional support for the client are extremely important during this stage. Relapse prevention efforts can include interactive discussions, role plays, and "what if" sessions in which the client identifies risks for relapse and develops workable strategies.

Revised from Bradley-Springer, 1996; sources: Grimley, DiClemente, Prochaska, & Prochaska, 1995; Prochaska, Redding, Harlow, Rossi, & Velicer, 1994.

behaviors and attitudes of provider, inability to develop meaningful relationships based on trust); lack of social support systems (including family relationships, available transportation, adequate housing, employment); abusive relationships; or problems with law enforcement. In addition, there are task-related & therapy factors that compound the problems such as lack of perceived benefits of therapy; lack of knowledge/understanding about the need for therapy; lack of knowledge/understanding about therapy and treatment protocols; complicated, long term, inconvenient treatment regimens; high degrees of required behavior change; changes that interfere with daily life; disturbing side effects (anticipated or actual); and behaviors (such as taking medications 3-6 times a day) that provide frequent and constant reminders of HIV (Britten, 1994; Crespo-Fiero, 1997; Klaus & Grodesky, 1997; Olfson, Hansell, & Boyer, 1997; Sowell, 1997).

HIV as a Chronic Disease

The complexity of HIV disease is, in many ways, related to its chronic nature. HIV-infected people share the problems experienced by all individuals with chronic diseases, but these problems are exacerbated by traumas related to the negative social constructs that surround HIV. Chronic diseases have no cure, continue for life, cause increasingly frequent periods of physical disability and dysfunction and ultimately contribute to morbidity and mortality. These rather dismal facts are compounded in a health care system, such as ours, that has difficulty dealing with chronicity and prefers to treat acute problems that respond rapidly to technological and chemical interventions (Thorne, 1993).

HIV infection leads to many of the consequences seen in other chronic diseases such as family stress, social isolation, dependence, frustration, lowered self-image, and economic pressures (Thorne, 1993). An interesting observation is that all of these variables may have contributed to the client's infection in the first place. Low self-esteem, searching for social contacts, frustration, and economic difficulties are all contributors to drug use and risky sexual behaviors.

Chronic diseases are characterized by acute exacerbations of intermittently developing problems that compound each other (Thorne, 1993). This is especially true in HIV disease where infections, cancers, debility, and social problems interact synergistically to tax the client's ability to cope. Physical deterioration in HIV disease is an erratic process. Instead of a steady, downward disease progression, HIV advances in an up and down manner. This is often confusing for nurses and clients as well as for families and significant others who all have difficulty dealing with the unpredictable, "good day/bad day" course of the disease. In addition, physical deterioration requires that the client deal with a body that no longer functions in the expected healthy manner. This breakdown in function and in the ability to depend on the body refocuses the client and decreases the ability to negotiate previously routine processes (Leonard, 1994). Chronic disease processes, especially those that develop in HIV infection, require the client to reassess bodily functions that can no longer be taken for granted. Instead, the client frequently becomes self-conscious and suspicious about the body's ability to respond as expected.

The major devastating problems associated with HIV include wasting, fatigue, diarrhea, pain, and dementia. These problems interact with a number of physical, psychosocial, and economic factors to create cycles of increasing illness. Wasting, for instance, is compounded for a client who is too tired to eat; has limited grocery money; has no social supports to help with meal preparation; rapidly loses nutritional intake through diarrhea or vomiting; has a malabsorption problem caused by HIV infection of the gastrointestinal (GI) tract; is too focused on mouth pain to care about eating; or has dementia-related symptoms that include forgetfulness and apathy. Wasting, in turn, worsens the fatigue, diarrhea, dementia, and economic situation. And poor nutritional status contributes to further deterioration of the immune system (Anastasi & Lee, 1994).

Chronic diseases are characterized by negative social constructs that stigmatize the client as being weak-willed or immoral for having the disease (Thorne, 1993). In HIV, this stigma is compounded by several factors. HIV-infected people are seen as lacking control over urges to have sex or use drugs. It is then easy to jump to the conclusion that they brought the disease on themselves and, therefore, somehow deserve to be sick. The behaviors associated with HIV infection are frequently viewed as immoral (homosexuality, multiple sex partners) and are sometimes illegal (drug use, prostitution). The fact that infected individuals can transmit the virus to others further entrenches the negative, stigmatizing social conception of HIV. Social stigmatization encourages discrimination in all facets of life. HIV-infected people have lost jobs, housing, and insurance because of such discrimination, even though this is illegal in the United States (The Americans with Disabilities Act, 1992 & 1994).

Holistic Nursing Care

The chronic nature of HIV disease requires the application of skilled nursing care that promotes a holistic view of the client. Holistic nursing care builds on the principles of prevention, health promotion, behavior change, and chronicity discussed above. Holistic care requires attention to all of the variables that could affect an individual client during his/her life with HIV infection. The nursing biopsychosocial approach to care is an ideal model for dealing with the complexities of HIV infection in a holistic and caring manner.

Humans are social animals and illness, especially chronic disease, disrupts social relationships (Thomasma, 1994). HIV is and has always been a family disease. Frequently, more than one member of the family is infected, but even if the disease is limited to one family member, the entire family becomes affected. An HIV-infected client's family may also be in need of nursing intervention. During the HIV epidemic, it has become even more evident that families exist in a variety of different structures. Some families consist of married couples and their children or married couples without children; some families include unmarried sexually-interacting couples of the same or opposite sex; some families include several generations while others have only one; and some families are simply a group of unrelated individuals who claim each other as family. The nurse must remember that the client defines her/his family. Peer and support group structures are equally important to consider when providing holistic care to HIV-infected individuals.

Cultural issues are of utmost importance when dealing with chronic disease. Each individual brings his/her personal constellation of cultures to the health care intervention. These cultures influence the client's actions in a number of ways, but because each client's constellation is unique, individualized assessment and interventions must be developed. HIV-infected clients will be influenced by their ethnic, religious, gender, age, sexual orientation, geographic, professional, socioeconomic, and familial cultures, to name a few.

All diseases occur in individuals with unique histories that have evolved through a lifetime of interactions within social, cultural, physical, and economic environments. In other words, each client must be approached within the context of his/her personal history; understanding cannot occur otherwise (Leonard, 1994). Because chronic disease assumes a major importance in the client's life, health care workers sometimes forget about the individual and focus instead on the disease. This is especially detrimental in HIV infection because of the stigmas discussed above. Holistic care requires an understanding of each client from a framework of past, present, and future possibilities. As one HIV-infected woman frequently says, "I am not HIV. I have a lot of other problems besides HIV and I have a life that continues despite HIV. HIV is only a part of who I am. It is not my life."

Thomasma (1994) has identified four levels of values that are important to the individual in search of health care. All of these values play into the client's decisions and life outcome. The levels, in ascending order of priority, are: *medical values,* which focus on organ systems and medically indicated procedures; the *therapeutic plan,* which delineates medical objectives and should take into consideration effects of treatment on the

client's life; *life plans* (the client's goals and future aspirations), which should guide the development of the therapeutic plan; and the client's *ultimate values* (the individual's guiding principles), which provide the basis for health care decisions.

HIV is best treated through a multidisciplinary team approach. The nurse frequently serves as the coordinator of the team, but it must be emphasized that the client is the most important team member. As possible, the client should serve as the team leader. Nursing advocacy can help to assure that this happens. The nursing care plan is actually a contractual agreement between the client and the nurse.

HIV care requires a wide variety of nursing interventions. Most nurses already possess the skills needed to provide appropriate care for HIV-infected individuals. Up-to-date information, positive attitudes, and clinical experience will increase the nurse's comfort and further insure that HIV-infected clients receive the best possible care.

Using this Book

The nursing diagnoses and interventions discussed in this book were selected after a review of a number of nursing texts (Carpenito, 1993; Daly, 1993; Flaskerud & Ungvarski, 1995; Grimes & Grimes, 1994; McFarland & McFarlane, 1993; Thompson, McFarland, Hirsch & Tucker, 1993). Carpenito's (1993) categorization system for nursing diagnoses is followed. This system is based on the North American Nursing Diagnosis Association (NANDA) taxonomy, but has additional features that are appealing to this author. Table 2.2 provides an overview of the selected nursing diagnoses that will be discussed in subsequent sections of the book. The following points will assist the nurse who uses this book:

Table 2.2. Nursing Diagnoses According to Prevention Level

CATEGORY	NURSING DIAGNOSIS[1]	1°	2°	3°	TD
Health Perception - Health Maintenance	Altered Health Maintenance	✔	✔		
	Health Seeking Behaviors		✔	✔	
	Ineffective Management of Therapeutic Regimen			✔	✔
	Noncompliance (Nonadherence)		✔	✔	
Nutritional - Metabolic	Hyperthermia			✔	✔
	Fluid Volume Deficit			✔	✔
	Fluid Volume Excess				✔
	Risk for Infection	✔		✔	DS
	Risk for Infection Transmission		✔	✔	✔
	Altered Nutrition: Less than Body Requirements			✔	✔
	Impaired Swallowing			✔	✔
	Impaired Skin Integrity			✔	DS
	Altered Oral Mucous Membranes			✔	✔
Elimination	Altered Bowel Elimination: Diarrhea			✔	✔
	Urinary Elimination: Functional Incontinence				✔
Activity-Exercise	Activity Intolerance			✔	DS
	Disuse Syndrome (Activity Intolerance, Risk for Infection, Risk for Injury, Impaired Physical Mobility, Powerlessness, Impaired Skin Integrity, Risk for Altered Respiratory Function, Body Image Disturbance, Sensory-Perceptual Alteration, Altered Tissue Perfusion, Constipation)				✔
	Impaired Home Maintenance Management			✔	✔
	Risk for Altered Respiratory Function			✔	DS
	Self-Care Deficit Syndrome (Bathing/Hygiene Self-Care Deficit, Dressing/Grooming Self-Care Deficit, Toileting Self-Care Deficit, Feeding Self-Care Deficit)				✔
	Instrumental Self-Care Deficit			✔	✔

[1]Classification according to Carpenito, L.J. (1993). *Handbook of Nursing Diagnosis* (5th ed.). Philadelphia: J.B. Lippincott Co.; TD indicates terminal disease, DS denotes incorporation into the diagnosis "Disuse Syndrome."

Table 2.2. Nursing Diagnoses According to Prevention Level

CATEGORY	NURSING DIAGNOSIS[1]	1°	2°	3°	TD
Sleep - Rest	Sleep Pattern Disturbance			✔	✔
Cognitive - Perceptual	Pain			✔	✔
	Decisional Conflict	✔	✔	✔	✔
	Sensory-Perceptual Alteration			✔	DS
	Altered Thought Process			✔	✔
Self-Perception	Anxiety		✔	✔	✔
	Fatigue		✔	✔	✔
	Fear	✔	✔	✔	✔
	Hopelessness		✔	✔	✔
	Powerlessness	✔	✔	✔	DS
	Body Image Disturbance			✔	DS
	Self-Esteem Disturbance	✔		✔	
	Chronic Low Self-Esteem	✔			
	Situational Low Self-Esteem		✔	✔	
Role-Relationship	Altered Family Processes	✔	✔	✔	✔
	Grieving			✔	✔
	Anticipatory Grieving		✔	✔	
	Dysfunctional Grieving			✔	✔
	Parental Role Conflict			✔	✔
	Impaired Social Interaction			✔	✔
	Social Isolation			✔	✔
Sexuality-Reproductive	Altered Sexuality Patterns	✔	✔	✔	✔
Coping-Stress Tolerance	Caregiver Role Strain			✔	✔
	Ineffective Individual Coping	✔	✔	✔	✔
	Ineffective Denial	✔	✔	✔	✔
	Ineffective Family Coping: Disabling			✔	✔
	Relocation Stress Syndrome			✔	✔
	Risk for Violence: Self-Directed		✔	✔	
Value-Belief	Spiritual Distress		✔	✔	✔

- The nursing diagnosis is always based on a nursing assessment. This book attempts to be comprehensive in the scope of possibly pertinent diagnoses; no client will need all of these diagnoses. Also, clients may have problems (such as diabetes mellitus or schizophrenia) that require additional diagnoses not discussed in the book.

- Nurses can manage a large number of the common problems in HIV infection through application of the nursing process. There are those problems, however, that require collaborative efforts of nurses and other health care providers including adverse medication reactions, electrolyte imbalance, encephalopathy, esophagitis, gastritis, hypovolemia, myelosuppression, meningitis, opportunistic disease, pneumonia, septicemia, and other sexually transmitted diseases (Carpenito, 1993). Other problems that may require collaborative efforts include psychological imbalances, social and financial difficulties, nutritional concerns, legal liabilities, spiritual impoverishment, speech and hearing deficits, occupational difficulties, mobility problems, etc.

- Nursing diagnoses may be actual or potential. Most can, therefore, be written with or without the phrase "at risk for . . ." Assessment will dictate whether the client requires interventions to prevent a problem ("at risk for . . .") or to prevent sequelae to a problem (actual diagnosis).

- Nursing diagnoses generally relate to otherwise healthy individuals. During some stages of HIV infection this is entirely possible. As clinical disease advances, however, people with HIV are more likely to have compounding physical, social, emotional, and economic problems that contribute to the complexity of the disease and nursing care problems.

- The nursing diagnosis, "Knowledge Deficit," is helpful only in the context of the situation where there is a problem related to a lack of information. Knowledge deficit is, therefore, not used in this book as an independent diagnosis, but is incorporated into other diagnoses as appropriate.

- All of the diagnoses discussed in this book require the following interventions. They are outlined here to decrease the amount of repetitious and overlapping information.

Interventions	Rationales
Develop a working knowledge of HIV infection, including transmission modes, risk reduction measures, signs and symptoms, medical treatment	Nurses are frequently the most readily available members of the health care team; being prepared with basic information to respond to client questions assists in the development of trust and establishes the nurse as a knowledgeable member of the health care team

Interventions	Rationales	Interventions	Rationales
Develop a trusting and supportive relationship with the client	Clients with HIV infection are often stigmatized and rejected by others in the community; the nurse-client relationship may be the most therapeutic interaction that is available to the client; the nurse provides optimal care if the relationship can endure long-term care demands; consistency and caring are high priorities for chronically ill clients	Involve family and significant others as much as possible if acceptable to the client	Reinforces the client's social support system; reassures significant others that they are an important part of the client's life; decreases confusion; gives others tasks that can increase their sense of being helpful and needed; assures the client that others will be there when needed; decreases the risk of others feeling left out and/or trying to sabotage health care interventions; helps client learn to accept assistance and care
Use touch with respect to personal comfort and cultural taboos; provide skin to skin contact (without gloves) between the nurse and the client as is comfortable for the client and in observation of BSI	Provides human contact; enhances the development of trust; demonstrates acceptance at a time when many feel unwanted and unloved; models safe and caring contact to family members and significant others; reinforces client self-esteem	Assure the client that confidentiality will be maintained	Because discrimination against HIV-infected people has led to a number of tragic consequences, confidentiality is even more important for the HIV-infected client than for others; insecurity about this issue may discourage HIV-infected people from seeking healthcare

Interventions	Rationales
Respect the client's individual context related to social, cultural, religious, and personal values	Individualized care provides the best chance for success; HIV-infected clients come with a history that includes all facets of their lives, not just the fact that they are infected with HIV
Employ a nonjudgmental approach to assessment and care	Behaviors that increase the risk of HIV are sometimes thought to be immoral and infected clients are frequently judged according to their risk factors; in fact, it doesn't matter *how* the client became infected, what matters is that s/he *is* infected and is in need of nursing care
Follow a philosophy of Harm Reduction that supports any and all steps, no matter how small, to decrease the risk of detrimental outcomes	Supports client in incremental steps toward safety and/or enhanced immune health; allows client to set personal pace and control life changes; successes at one level encourage initiation of changes at higher, more difficult levels

Interventions	Rationales
Use the Transtheoretical Model to assess status and determine interventions that help clients make positive health changes throughout the course of the disease	Provides a consistent approach to behavior change that focuses on the individual client's current status in the cycle of change; provides encouragement at all stages of change; acknowledges client right to self-determination
Use appropriate humor	Defuses difficult situations; makes health care more tolerable; communicates acceptance; enhances the nurse-client relationship; decreases stress; reinforces commitment to holistic care; meets socialization needs
Respect the client's right to make decisions about personal health issues	There are still unanswered questions in the treatment of HIV disease and treatment decisions are always laden with uncertainty; decisions must be based on current knowledge and evaluated according to personal values; nurses assist this process, but do not make the ultimate decisions; empowered clients are more motivated to become involved in health-seeking behaviors

Interventions	Rationales	Interventions	Rationales
Honor the need of human beings to find meaning in the events and circumstances of their lives	Searching for meaning is an attempt to make sense of life problems; meaning is generally related to a person's level of comfort and harmony with the self, family, significant others, and a spiritual base that may be described as a higher power; relationship and spiritual explorations during the progression of HIV disease are not unusual	View HIV as a community problem that can be approached in various community, education, religious, political, and economic settings; provide up-to-date information to community leaders; interact with community-based organizations to improve care and services for HIV-infected clients, their families, and significant others; lobby for health care reforms, anti-discrimination laws, and improved funding for HIV-related issues; educate citizens of all ages to prevent transmission of HIV and to increase compassion for those already infected	Prevention and discrimination issues must be addressed in public arenas in order to get information to all facets of society; nurses have knowledge and skills to disseminate appropriate information to communities

Chapter III

Primary Prevention

Primary prevention interventions are appropriate for clients who are not currently infected with HIV. Primary prevention is an important public health strategy that, when successful, has the ability to significantly decrease morbidity and mortality. Every disease that is prevented represents a savings in human suffering and health care costs. Every case of HIV that is prevented represents a break in the chain of disease-transmission-infection-disease. The goals of primary prevention in HIV infection are to:

1. Prevent infection.
2. Promote risk reduction activities.

In the absence of a vaccination, education and behavior change are the only effective tools for prevention of HIV.

Primary prevention measures should take place in all health care, educational, and social settings because everyone needs to know the basics about HIV infection and AIDS. Knowledge and skill development assist with the goals of primary prevention by reinforcing information and helping people who are at low or no risk to maintain that status. Knowledgeable individuals have the ability to question new activities, evaluate risk, make choices that decrease potential risks, and use equipment and communication skills in an effective manner. Table 1.1 provides a quick review of safe, risk reducing, and high risk activities. See Introduction for a more detailed discussion.

Primary prevention measures should be addressed to communities as well as to individuals because it is often the community that supports or ignores problems that increase the risk of exposure to HIV. Nurses must be willing to share their expertise in the areas of assessment, community organization, education, and political activism. Some of the areas that need this attention include:

sexually transmitted disease; drug use; family violence; teen pregnancy; gang activity; gender discrimination; and acceptance of cultural, social, racial, and sexual orientation differences.

Risk Assessment

People who are already involved in behaviors that put them at risk for HIV infection need to have more focused prevention interventions. Nurses can help clients assess their risks by asking some very basic questions. In the Risk Assessment Interview (below), the bold type questions are the minimum needed to initiate an assessment for risk of HIV infection. Questions should be modified to meet the needs of the client and the situation. Positive responses to any of these questions require an in-depth exploration of the issues, as represented in the follow-up questions.

Risk Assessment Interview

Climate setting tips:

- Arrange for the interview to take place in a comfortable, quiet, private setting.

- Introduce yourself and provide information about your job and responsibilities.

- Assess client's emotional state and relieve anxiety as much as possible.

- Acknowledge that the interview will deal with sensitive issues. A possible way to accomplish this is to say, "I'm going to be asking you some very personal questions. I would not ask them if it didn't make a difference in your health care. How you answer the questions will help us to discuss what you can do to stay healthy."

- Assure confidentiality of information.

- Start with the least sensitive questions before progressing to more personal issues.

Questions	Rationales
Have you ever had a transfusion or used clotting factor? If yes: Were you using clotting factor before 1985? How often did you use clotting factor before 1985? Is your hemophilia considered to be mild, moderate, or severe?	Clotting factor has been heat or chemically treated since 1985 to prevent transmission of HIV and HBV; risk is greater for severe hemophiliacs who tend to use factor more often
How many transfusions have you had? Were any of the transfusions before 1985? What were the circumstances? Where were you when you had the transfusion?	The more transfusions, the greater the risk; risk of infection from transfusion after 1985 (when testing was initiated) is very low; communities and countries with high prevalence levels of HIV increase the risk for transfusion recipients, especially before 1985; testing blood for HIV is not done routinely in many countries, especially those that are not considered to be "developed" nations

Questions	Rationales
Have you ever had an accidental exposure to blood? If so, what was the route of exposure - to skin, mucous membranes or through a puncture wound?	Risk is highest through puncture wounds; exposure to intact skin and mucous membranes creates significantly less risk
Was the blood known to be HIV infected? Did it come from a person who was at high risk for HIV infection?	HIV cannot be transmitted in the blood of an uninfected person; review client records to determine if HIV testing has been done and to assess client's risk factors
What, if any, follow up did you receive after the exposure(s)?	Helps determine the client's knowledge of post-exposure follow up; allows assessment of emotional state related to exposure
Have you ever shared needles, syringes, or other injection equipment (works) with anyone? If yes: Do you still inject drugs? If so, what do you inject and how often? Do you still share your works?	Assesses continuing risk and current drug using behaviors

Questions	Rationales	Questions	Rationales
Have any of the people with whom you shared developed HIV infection or AIDS?	Although client may not know this, it can provide information about degree of risk	If you still inject drugs: What do you inject? Do you share injection equipment (works)? How often do you share? With whom do you share? Where do you get your equipment? What, if anything, do you do to decrease your risks when injecting drugs? Do you clean your equipment? If so, how? when? Do you use other drugs (such as marijuana or alcohol) that are not injected? Have you ever quit using? Do you want to quit?	Provides drug use history that can help establish risk and provide basis for education about risk reduction measures and/or treatment options; gives input on knowledge and current practices used to decrease risk
If you no longer inject drugs: When was the last time you injected? Where were you living? When was the last time that you shared equipment?	Seroprevalence rates of HIV in drug users differ from community to community and over time; higher prevalence rates increase risk of transmission		
What were you injecting? Are you now drug free? If not, what do you use and how do you use it?	Provides drug use history that can help in developing strategies to prevent relapse; assesses current drug use and allows for reinforcements of risk reducing behaviors (i.e., smoking, but not injecting, heroin); establishes need for further education related to sexual experiences while "high"	Have you ever had a blackout as a result of using drugs? Have you ever had sex while under the influence of drugs?	Helps to establish possible sexual risks while using; these questions refer to any drug taken by any route, including alcohol, marijuana, narcotics, and street drugs

Questions	Rationales
Have you ever had a sexual experience in which your penis, vagina, rectum, or mouth came into contact with another person's penis, vagina, rectum, or mouth? If yes: Do you have, or have you ever had sex with men, women, or both?	A nonjudgmental way of discovering historical information about sexuality; risk is higher for gay men in some communities where prevalence rates are high among homosexuals; however, risk is present for all sexually active individuals
Do you have, or have you ever had, vaginal, oral, anal sex, or all three? (Client may need a definition of one or all of these.)	A nonjudgmental way of discovering information about sexual practices; sets stage for discussions about safe, risk reducing, and high-risk practices
Do you have, or have you ever had, sexual contact with a person who was known to have HIV infection or AIDS? Do you have, or have you ever had, sexual contact with a person who was known to be at high risk for HIV infection or AIDS?	People who know or suspect a partner's HIV status have special needs for support, education, and skill development

Questions	Rationales
Have you ever had a sexually transmitted disease?	Establishes a history of sexual risk
Have you ever exchanged sex for money or drugs?	Sexual activities under these circumstances provide additional safety and infection risks
How many sexual partners have you had since 1981? in the past year? in the past month?	This may be a less important issue than in the past, but it can still help establish degree of risk, especially for individuals living in high-incidence areas
Are you worried about any of your sexual relationships? If so, why?	Individuals may have suspicions about the infection status of sexual partners; these suspicions may provide motivation for testing and/or behavior change
What methods, if any, do you use to protect yourself during sexual activity?	Nonjudgmental method of introducing topic of protection related to barriers, partner selection, use of nonpenetrative sex

Clients who are assessed to be at risk for HIV infection need to have appropriate education and counseling. Educational messages should be specific to the client's need, culturally sensitive, and age specific. An emphasis should be placed on skill development (i.e., negotiating skills, condom use, and cleaning used injection equipment) and access to resources. Individuals at high risk of being infected with HIV should be encouraged to get tested (see Secondary Prevention).

Specific Nursing Diagnoses and Interventions

Altered Health Maintenance

A state in which an individual is at risk of becoming infected with HIV because of risky behaviors. The individual has a desire to change risky behaviors in order to maintain uninfected status but requires assistance to identify, manage, or seek help for behavior change.

Related to:

Lack of knowledge; misunderstanding of information; ineffective coping; lack of access to healthcare, health education, or drug treatment services; lack of access to equipment (condoms, sterile injection equipment)

Defining Characteristics:

Unhealthy or risky behaviors

- **Subjective Findings:** Acknowledges unhealthy practices, especially those involving substance use and high-risk sexual behaviors; verbalizes desire to change risky behavior

- **Objective Findings:** Substance use, history of STDs; knowledge, and/or skills deficits

Outcome criteria:

Reduced risk of infection with HIV

Interventions	Rationales
Help the client identify a specific goal for change	Reinforces motivation and clarifies desired final outcome
Assess the client's current level of knowledge and skill in relation to the desired change; determine knowledge and skill deficits	Provides information about where education and skill development interventions need to start
Explore the spectrum of safe, risk reducing, and high-risk behaviors; determine practices that are acceptable for the client	Helps client determine acceptable course based on preference and ability, as well as social, cultural, religious, and family norms
Encourage movement toward safer activities by asking client, "What is safer than what you are currently doing? Is that something that would work for you? If not, what is safer and possible for you?"	Safe activities, especially abstinence, are often not acceptable choices; pointing out risk reducing activities that are safer and more palatable starts the process of incremental change

Interventions	Rationales
Assist with identifying incremental steps in achieving the goal	Divides the larger goal into achievable bits, making the task less overwhelming and improving the chance of success
Provide continuing support that encourages incremental behavior change; remind client that consistent change takes time and effort; remind client that relapse is not failure and that protective behaviors can be re-initiated	Behavior change occurs over time and may have periods of relapse; continuing support gives client positive input and encourages continued efforts; identifying even small successes encourages continuation of effort
As possible, include family and/or significant others in behavior change planning and support process	Changes in sexual or drug using behaviors also affect the client's significant others who may be threatened by the desired change, may not want the client to change, or may be tempted to sabotage the process; support from significant others, on the other hand, is a powerful motivator for behavior change
Explore other potential barriers to desired behavior change	There may be limited access to treatment programs, support groups, necessary equipment, etc.; the client may lack necessary social skills

Interventions	Rationales
Determine resources and referrals that will assist the client to overcome potential barriers and sustain change efforts	Community-based HIV organizations, social service providers, HIV-dedicated clinical treatment facilities, and drug treatment centers may be able to provide the support needed to sustain behavior change efforts through counseling, education, support groups, condom distribution, syringe and needle exchange, drug treatment, etc.

Evaluation:

The client:

1. Lists alternatives to risky behaviors
2. Demonstrates knowledge and skills that are necessary for behavior change
3. Verbalizes intent to change risky behaviors
4. Initiates a plan for behavior change
5. Reports behavior changes over time

Risk for Infection

A state in which an individual is at increased risk for being infected with HIV.

Related to:

A history of transfusion or use of clotting factor; a history of sharing equipment for injecting drugs; a history of unprotected sexual intercourse with HIV-infected partners, or partners whose HIV status was not known; an accidental exposure to HIV-infected blood, semen, or vaginal secretions.

Defining Characteristics:

Involvement in risk producing behaviors

- **Subjective Findings:** Identifies personal risky behaviors; expresses concern about risk

- **Objective Findings:** History of other STDs; injection (track) marks on skin (may appear on arms, hands, legs, feet, neck, or breasts); immune suppression related to substance use (tobacco, alcohol, street drugs)

Outcome criteria:

Prevention of HIV infection

Interventions	Rationales
Assess level of risk	Establishes need for further intervention; provides opportunity to allay fears in those at low risk
Determine source of risk	Education and prevention messages must be based on individual client need, for instance, education after a needle stick exposure differs from education needed by a client with a history of continuing drug use

Interventions	Rationales
Teach client how to avoid infection: be specific to his/her risk and provide practice sessions for equipment use (i.e., condoms), equipment care (i.e., cleaning used works), and communication skills (i.e., negotiating condom use, saying "no," gaining social support to leave unsafe relationship)	Provides specific, immediately applicable education that is more useful to the client and, therefore, more likely to be used; also see interventions for Altered Health Maintenance (above)
Refer for testing and counseling if risk assessment indicates need	If client is already HIV infected, nursing care moves into secondary prevention

Evaluation:

The client:

1. Remains free from HIV infection
2. Demonstrates knowledge and skills required to remain free of HIV infection

Decisional Conflict

A state of indecision between competing choices that involve risk, loss, or challenge to established personal lifestyle or values.

*Author's Note:

Deciding to change to less risky sex or drug using behaviors can result in serious personal and/or interpersonal conflicts and may lead to more immediate risks such as abandonment or physical or sexual abuse (see Fear, below).

Related to:

Confusing, inconsistent, or incomplete information related to prevention of HIV infection; disagreement within support system about best course to take; inexperience in decision making; unclear personal value system, or a conflict with personal values; ethical dilemmas related to sexuality or drug use; lack of information about alternatives

Defining Characteristics:

Inability to decide on course of action

- **Subjective Findings:** Verbalizes uncertainty; worries about negative consequences of perceived choices; recognizes increased stress; questions value system

- **Objective Findings:** Vacillation between choices; delayed decision making; behaviors that are counter to expressed goals

Outcome Criteria:

Informed decisions that work for the client

Interventions	Rationales
Assist client to identify the problem, explore options, list positive and negative attributes of each option, identify probable outcomes for each option, and evaluate each option for compatibility with personal values, lifestyle, and support system; reassure client that he or she can make the decision and has the right to do so	Clarifies problem and encourages a thoughtful progression toward a decision that is acceptable to the client; empowers the client to make own decision with support as needed

Interventions	Rationales
If acceptable to the client, encourage involvement of family and significant others in decision making process	Assures others that they remain an important part of the client's life; helps others buy into a supportive position
Actively support client's decision even if it is not the decision you would make; ascertain that client understands all components of the decision, including potential negative consequences	Reinforces client's right to make decisions; demonstrates that decisions will not be undermined; provides assurance that client is aware of potential problems
Initiate teaching to decrease knowledge and skill deficits (see Altered Health Maintenance and Risk of Infection above)	Provides knowledge and skills to implement choices that decrease risk

Evaluation:

The client:

1. Realistically states advantages and disadvantages of each option
2. Discusses fears and concerns about options
3. Weighs options and comes to an informed choice
4. Acquires knowledge and skill to implement choices
5. Expresses satisfaction with choice

Fear

A state in which the client experiences a feeling of dread related to decisions to make changes toward less risky behaviors. The source of the fear is identifiable and perceived to be dangerous.

Related to:

Possibility of HIV infection; potential consequences of behavior change: loss of status or place in peer group; rejection of family or significant others; disruption of lifestyle; withdrawal; physical or emotional abuse

Defining Characteristics:

Lack of action related to fear of outcomes

- **Subjective Findings:** Discusses feelings of dread, fright and apprehension; verbal reports of panic or obsession

- **Objective Findings:** Avoidance behaviors; narrow focus on danger; reactive behaviors such as crying, aggression, hypervigilance, compulsive activities, and escapism; anger; reassurance seeking behaviors

Outcome Criteria:

Decreased fear, comfort with choosing alternatives

Interventions	Rationales
Seek to understand client's perspective of fear inducing situations: encourage expression of feelings; solicit realistic descriptions of fearful situations and threatening individuals	Establishes a relationship in which the client feels safe discussing fearful situations; encourages client to base fears on past experience or realistic expectations; enhances development of empathy
Assess risk and provide for client safety as a first priority	Compromises may have to be made to keep client safe and/or alive; for instance, it may be safer for a woman to not insist on condom use if her male partner becomes violent when it is mentioned; instead, discuss with her the possibilities of getting out of the abusive relationship (an action that may be equally or even more frightening)
Assist client in decision making: assess decision making ability, discourage decision making during periods of high stress; also see Decisional Conflict (above)	Assures thoughtful process and discourages hasty, nonprotective decisions; empowers client to take responsibility for personal life

Interventions	Rationales
Make appropriate referrals for social and economic support	Discussing issues with professionals and/or people in similar situations clarifies fear and helps client explore options; financial support can assist client who feels "stuck" in a bad situation

Evaluation:

The client:

1. Identifies acceptable personal coping mechanisms that are judged to be effective
2. Verbalizes feelings of increased safety

Powerlessness

A state in which the client perceives a lack of personal control over ability to prevent infection with HIV.

Related to:

Lack of knowledge; dependence on peer group, family, or significant others; feelings of inevitability based on history of drug use and/or sexual activity; life experiences that reinforce lack of control

Defining Characteristics:

Lack of ability to exert personal choice

- **Subjective Findings:** Expresses discomfort or hostility over inability to control situation; verbalizes concerns about lack of control over outcome

- **Objective Findings:** Behaviors and attitudes that indicate dissatisfaction with lack of power such as: apathy, aggression, acting-out behaviors, anxiety, depression, resignation, passive-aggressive behaviors; nonparticipation in therapeutic interventions

Outcome Criteria:

Increased sense of personal control

Interventions	Rationales
Encourage client to talk about feelings, perceptions and fears related to assuming personal responsibility	Helps client realize the extent to which others influence her/his life
Discuss HIV-related consequences of allowing others to control life	Demonstrates dependency on others to decrease risk of infection and dangers inherent in not having personal control
Encourage client to take as much personal responsibility for staying uninfected with HIV as possible	Includes aspects of Altered Health Maintenance, Risk for Infection, Decisional Conflict, and Fear (see above)
Help client determine areas where it is safe, comfortable, or feasible to exert more control; assist with development of plan to assume more control in these areas	Helps client practice in situations where there is a good chance of success

Interventions	Rationales
Monitor progress and provide positive feedback for appropriate use of power	Decreases the likelihood of relapse; helps client return to behavior after relapse

Evaluation:

The client:

1. Identifies control issues that are stressful
2. Realistically assesses factors that can be controlled by self
3. Makes and follows through on decisions

Self-Esteem Disturbance

A state of negative self-evaluation about self- or personal capability.

*Author's Note:

Lack of self-esteem increases the risk of drug use and risky sexual behaviors because these can temporarily enhance self-image, feelings of worth, and feelings of being accepted while dulling feelings of inferiority and rejection.

Related to:

Sexual abuse; relationship problems; loss of a relationship; failure in school or at work; ineffective relationships with parents/ parental rejection; history of abusive relationships; unrealistic expectations of self; abuse of drugs or alcohol by self or family; co-dependency issues; legal difficulties; negative social or cultural influences that discriminate according to gender, race, age, or sexual orientation

Defining Characteristics:

Poor self-image

- **Subjective Findings:** Makes self-negating comments; expresses guilt or shame; evaluates self as incapable, inferior, or inadequate; denies problems; discusses feelings of lack of power or control; verbalizes problems with gender and/or sexual identity

- **Objective Findings:** Self-negating behaviors; indecisiveness; inability to set goals or make decisions; poor problem solving skills; signs of depression; self-abusive behaviors (including substance use, sexually acting-out behavior, and assuming the role of victim); projecting blame and responsibility to others; hesitancy to respond or initiate actions; poor eye contact

Outcome Criteria:

Enhanced self-esteem

Interventions	Rationales
Explore self-perception issues with client in a non-judgmental manner: examine negative perceptions; analyze impact of others on self-esteem; discuss reasons for self-criticism or guilt; identify significance of issues (such as age, gender, sexual orientation, culture, religion, etc.) that influence self-esteem	Provides opportunities for understanding where negative self-image comes from; demonstrates acceptance of client despite litany of negative factors; reinforces self-worth

Interventions	Rationales
Discuss ways in which personal self-concept influences risk of HIV infection: using risky behaviors to establish self as part of group, as a coping mechanism, or a substitute for meaningful social relationships	Helps client realize the risk that acceptance-seeking behaviors create; provides opportunity to move on to discussions of risk reduction measures and referrals to support groups
Explore client's positive attributes and accomplishments: identify strengths, point out attractive physical features, reinforce past accomplishments	Reinforces presence of positive attributes; enhances self-esteem
Recommend activities that show and reinforce personal capabilities: encourage realistic goal setting, increased responsibility, self-evaluation, and social interaction; encourage activities that contribute to or support others, increase social interactions and enhance physical capabilities	Provides external source of esteem that may become internalized as successes accumulate

Interventions	Rationales
Identify underlying cause and initiate appropriate treatment or referrals	Some deep-seated causes of low self-esteem such as physical or sexual abuse, drug use, parental neglect, or overt discrimination require specialized treatment and counseling

Evaluation:

The client:

1. Discusses self-perceptions
2. Realistically analyzes personal capabilities
3. Reflects on positive personal attributes

Chronic Low Self-Esteem

A state of longstanding problems related to self-esteem.

*Author's Note:

This creates a particularly high risk for HIV infection. People who feel that they are worthless are more likely to become involved in risk behaviors that provide temporary solace, but ultimately lead to increased self-esteem problems.

Related to:

History of repeated internal and external insults to self-worth, related to any or all of the factors listed in Self-Esteem Disturbance (above)

Defining Characteristics:

Longstanding or chronic self-image problem

- **Subjective Findings:** Discusses over-dependency on others; makes statements that negate self-worth

- **Objective Findings:** Frequent lack of success in personal and work life; body language, personal hygiene, and/or grooming denote poor self-image; passivity; indecisiveness; excessive need for reassurance

Outcome Criteria:

Enhanced self-esteem

Interventions	Rationales
Implement interventions outlined in Self-Esteem Disturbance (above)	Initiates assessment and care
Encourage social interactions and situations in which new skills can be practiced	Successful interactions can enhance self-esteem and reinforce new skills
Set limits for problem behaviors, including self-recrimination/blame, aggression, and preoccupation with death/suicide	Acknowledges that these problems may exist; helps client identify triggers and alternatives to these behaviors
Discuss vocational interests and develop plans to pursue job/educational opportunities	Ability to support self is self-affirming, reinforces capability, and promotes independence
Provide appropriate reading materials if desired by client	Supports and reinforces information for those who use this learning style

Interventions	Rationales
Refer for long-term counseling	Enhances chance of dealing with longstanding image problem

Evaluation:

The client:

1. Develops more realistic expectations of self
2. Lists positive attributes
3. Moves toward less risky behaviors
4. Moves toward healthier, more assertive social interactions

Altered Family Processes

A state in which a family that normally functions effectively experiences a stressor that challenges functional status.

Related to:

Individual family member's desire to change behaviors that are perceived to be risky (families are often intimately involved in sexual or drug using activities); disruption of family routines; change in role of a family member; breach of trust among members related to discovery/change of sexual activity or drug use

Defining Characteristics:

Family system experiences difficulty in adapting to changes

- **Subjective Findings:** Client and/or family members discuss feelings of discomfort within family; client verbalizes need to find other sources of support and/or makes statements such as, "I love my family, but they just don't understand me anymore," or "I just can't talk to my wife/husband/partner anymore!"

- **Objective Findings:** Communication problems develop within family; physical, emotional, spiritual, or safety needs of individual no longer met by family; history of long-term problems within family of origin

Outcome Criteria:

Improved understanding and coping ability within family

Interventions	Rationales
Identify conflicts among family members: individuals who suddenly refuse to share injection equipment or insist on using condoms create suspicion and anxiety, change the structure of the family, disrupt roles within the family, and threaten family stability	Provides insight to all family members about what is happening to the individual and how this is affecting the family; provides basis for further discussion and problem solving; recognizes that most people desire positive relationships with the family of origin

Interventions	Rationales
Assist family to resolve conflict: use problem-solving skills; encourage expressions of guilt, hostility and anger; build on past family caring cohesiveness, and support; refer to family therapy as appropriate	Helps family members identify real issues ("You think I have AIDS, don't you?"; "If you're too good to share my works then you're too good to share my drugs."; "Condoms give me a rash."); facilitates interactions that can lead to positive change; defuses potentially volatile situations
Provide continuing support to individual within family who desires change to decrease risk of HIV	Ultimate concern is to prevent new cases of HIV infection; successful changes by one family member may influence positive change in others

Evaluation:

Family members:

1. Verbalize concerns about family function
2. Communicate concerns to other family members
3. Maintain support system for all family members
4. Resolve issues, remembering that one form of resolution is to peacefully and safely dissolve the family unit

Altered Sexuality Patterns

A state in which an individual expresses concerns about any aspect of sexual function or sexual health.

Related to:

Desire to develop less risky sexual interactions; fear of infection with HIV; development or fear of other sexually transmitted diseases

Defining Characteristics:

Anxiety about sexual function if less risky sexual activities are incorporated

- **Subjective Findings:** Describes actual or anticipated changes in sexual function or sexual identity in light of plans to initiate less risky practices; expresses concern about sexuality; verbalizes concern about partner's acceptance of changes

- **Objective Findings:** Anxiety; fear; vacillations about decisions to initiate changes to increase safety

Outcome Criteria:

Comfortable sexual function while reducing risks

Interventions	Rationales
Assess sexual history (see Risk Assessment Interview above): encourage holistic exploration of personal issues that affect sexual function	Provides basis for care plan and development of interventions; demonstrates that sex is an acceptable topic; reinforces that sexuality is an important component of the client's life and health; sexuality is influenced by a wide variety of factors, any one of which can create potential barriers to behavior change

Interventions	Rationales
Provide reassurance and encourage experimentation in alternate forms of sexual expression; provide "practice sessions": simulate client-partner verbal communications and negotiations in role plays; develop condom use skills with dildos or cucumbers to simulate an erect penis; develop female condom use skills with plastic models of the vagina	Decreases inhibitions that can limit client's willingness to expand choices in sexual expression; decreases anxiety; provides support in a safe environment
Use appropriate humor and encourage client to use humor as a way of relieving embarrassment	Acknowledges that sexuality is a sensitive issue; sends message that sexual activity can/should be an enjoyable, fun, healthy experience
Implement care as outlined in Altered Health Maintenance, Decisional Conflict, Fear, Powerlessness, Self-Esteem Disturbance, and Chronic Low Self-Esteem (above)	All of these issues influence sexuality and ability to change current level of sexual function

Evaluation:

The client:

1. Discusses concerns about sexuality
2. Develops strategies for sexual interactions that decrease current level of risk for HIV
3. Verbalizes satisfaction with sexual function

Ineffective Individual Coping

A state in which an individual experiences an inability to adapt, solve problems, or manage everyday stressors because of inadequate resources.

Related to:

Disruptions of relationships; poverty; inadequate support system; low self-esteem; stress overload; persistent social/cultural oppression

Defining Characteristics:

Inadequate coping capabilities

- **Subjective Findings:** Verbalizes feelings of inability to cope with situations related to the risk of HIV infection and/or the problems caused by desire to change behaviors to decrease risk

- **Objective Findings:** Inability to initiate change; lack of follow-up to resource referrals; impaired self-concept; poor problem-solving skills; impaired communication skills

Outcome Criteria:

Enhanced coping abilities

Interventions	Rationales
Implement care as outlined in Altered Health Maintenance, Decisional Conflict, Fear, Powerlessness, Self-Esteem Disturbance, Chronic Low Self-Esteem, and Altered Family Processes	All of these issues influence coping ability
Work within the community to develop effective programs that support community organization and social change	Initiates efforts to decrease stereotypes, discrimination, and oppression (above)
Help client identify stressors that cannot be dealt with directly; explore stress reducing practices that help with generalized stress reduction such as exercise, yoga, meditation, relaxation techniques	Identifies problems that the client cannot control; reinforces ability to care for self despite lack of power in these areas
Ask client to describe previous encounters with stressor; encourage client to critique encounters to discover helpful and less helpful coping strategies	Allows reflection; encourages development of new coping methods that can be applied to future confrontations; reinforces assurance that positive coping can occur

Interventions	Rationales
Refer to support groups, counselors, or others who have an understanding of the client's situational stressors	Provides a network of knowledgeable individuals who can provide situation-specific support and guidance

Evaluation:

The client:

1. Discusses issues that appear to be overwhelming
2. Identifies resources that can provide support
3. Develops coping plan and follows through with appropriate actions

Ineffective Denial

A state in which an individual consciously or unconsciously attempts to disavow a risk of HIV infection in order to reduce anxiety or fear.

Related to:

Inability to acknowledge risk of becoming infected with HIV; knowledge deficit; low self-esteem; feelings of inadequacy, guilt, loneliness, despair, failure, anger, frustration, anxiety

Defining Characteristics:

Inability to accept risk of being infected with HIV

- **Subjective Findings:** Verbalizes feelings of anxiety; denies HIV has personal relevancy; denies vulnerability or responsibility related to HIV infection

- **Objective Findings:** Refuses to seek information to the detriment of health; does not perceive dangers inherent in denial (for self or others); minimizes risk; stress symptoms

Outcome Criteria:

Acknowledges risk for HIV infection

Interventions	Rationales
Determine basis for denial	Provides important assessment information that may lead to focused interventions such as those described above in Risk for Infection, Decisional Conflict, Fear, Powerlessness, Self-Esteem Disturbance, Chronic Low Self-Esteem, Altered Family Processes, and Altered Sexuality Patterns
Avoid direct confrontation of denial	Reduces risk of entrenching denial; prevents destruction of therapeutic relationship
Explore client's interpretation of the situation: history of risk, knowledge of HIV	Reduces risk of entrenching denial; prevents destruction of therapeutic relationship

Interventions	Rationales
Use a focus of protecting the client to initiate risk reduction discussions	Encourages client to learn and use safe or risk reducing behaviors that will protect others in the community; see Primary Prevention
Correct inaccuracies and deficiencies in knowledge base	Clarifies information and limits use of erroneous information as basis for denial

Evaluation:

The client:

1. Identifies fears and anxieties related to HIV infection
2. Protects self from exposure to HIV
3. Develops a knowledge base that supports acceptance of risk
4. Implements alternative coping strategies
5. Experiences reduction in fear and/or anxiety

Chapter IV

Secondary Prevention

An individual who is infected with HIV but still asymptomatic will require care at the secondary prevention level; most of the care at this point is provided on an out-patient basis. Nursing care focuses on detection of HIV and early intervention. The goals of care are to:

1. Detect HIV infection as early as possible
2. Promote health and limit disability
3. Assist with and support decisions around treatment options
4. Promote adjustment to chronic disease
5. Prevent further transmissions of HIV
6. Keep client involved in the health care system

Detection of HIV infection is based on risk assessment (see Primary Prevention), recognition of early signs and symptoms (see Introduction), and testing (see Introduction). Testing for HIV infection is an important part of the public health response to HIV and the only effective method for determining if an individual is actually infected. People who are at risk of being infected with HIV should be encouraged to be tested. All testing for HIV should be accompanied by pre- and post-test counseling (see below) that provides opportunities for risk assessment, education, and development of a therapeutic relationship.

Community efforts at the secondary prevention level continue to focus on education. Nurses who know about HIV-testing practices and sites in their communities can provide valuable information to individuals and groups through public forums and mass media. Nurses can also assist communities by educating to decrease HIV-related knowledge deficiencies that may contribute to attitudes that promote discrimination against HIV-infected individuals.

Some clinicians now recommend initiation of antiretroviral therapy (ART) as early as possible in HIV infection (see Introduction). Because this is not a universally agreed-upon intervention, however, care must be taken to help clients understand their various choices. Some clients, especially those in rural areas, will need assistance in finding knowledgeable care providers who are comfortable with the various options now offered by multidrug therapy. Others will need assistance in finding care providers who support individual choices in treatment.

Guides for Pre- and Post-Test Counseling

General Guidelines

- People who are being tested for HIV are usually fearful about the test results.

- Establish rapport with the client.

- Assess client's ability to understand counseling.

- Determine the client's ability to access support systems.

- Discuss the following methods of testing that are available in most states:

  - *Confidential testing* requires that the client give her or his name, address, and phone number. The lab slip and blood are labeled in a way that allows for the results to be matched with the named individual. This may occur during the process (the name goes on the lab slip and the test tube) or may only occur when the results come back to the clinician (a number or other identifier is placed on the lab slip and test tube). Test results are treated like other information that appears on a client's chart: Health care providers are ethically required to keep all such information confidential.

- *Anonymous testing* preserves the anonymity of the client because no identifying information is required. The client is given a number that is also attached to the lab slip and test tube. Results are disclosed only when the client presents the number at the test site. This system encourages testing in those individuals who are fearful that their test status will be disclosed to others who may seek to harm the client in some way. The disadvantage is that the client is required to complete the process by returning for results. Non-returners cannot be contacted.

- Explain the benefits of testing:

  - Testing provides an opportunity for education that can decrease the risk of new infections.
  - Infected individuals can be referred for early intervention and support programs.
  - Testing can relieve the anxiety related to not knowing an HIV infection status.

- Discuss negative aspects of testing:

  - Confidentiality issues: Breeches of confidentiality have led to discrimination.
  - A positive test affects all aspects of the client's life (personal, social, economic, etc.) and can raise difficult emotional issues such as anger, anxiety, guilt, and thoughts of suicide.

Pre-Test Counseling

- Determine the client's risk factors and when the last risk occurred (see Risk Assessment in Primary Prevention).

Counseling should be individualized according to these parameters.

- Provide education to decrease future risk of exposure.

- Provide education that will help the client protect sex and drug using partners.

- Discuss problems related to the delay between infection and an accurate test. Testing will need to be done up to 6 months after each possible exposure. Discuss the continuing need to abstain from or decrease risk behaviors. Discuss the need to protect sex and drug using partners during that interval.

- Discuss the possibility of false negative tests, which are most likely to occur during the window period (up to 6 months after initial infection).

- Explain that a positive test shows *HIV infection,* not AIDS. AIDS must be diagnosed according to criteria established by the CDC (see Introduction).

- Explain that the test *does not establish immunity,* regardless of the results. There is currently no known immune state for HIV.

- Assess support systems. Provide lists of local telephone numbers and resources, as needed.

- Ask client, "What will you do if your HIV test is positive?" and "What will you do if your HIV test is negative?"

- Outline assistance that will be offered if the test is positive.

Post-Test Counseling

- If the test is negative, reinforce pre-test counseling and prevention education. Remind client that the test needs to be repeated 6 months after the most recent exposure risk. If less than 6 months has elapsed since last possible exposure to HIV, reinforce information about protecting sex and drug using partners.

- If the test is positive, understand that the client may be in shock and not hear much of what you say.

  - Provide resources for medical and emotional support and help the client get immediate assistance.
  - Evaluate suicide risk and follow up as needed.
  - Determine need to test others who have had risky contact with the client. Solicit client's cooperation in identifying contacts. Initiate contact with the Health Department so that contact tracing can begin.
  - Discuss retesting to verify results. This tactic supports hope for the client, but more importantly, keeps the client in the system. While waiting for the second test result, the client has time to think about and adjust to the possibility of being HIV infected.
  - Encourage optimism:
    - Remind client that treatments are available.
    - Review health habits that can improve immune function.
    - Arrange for client to speak to HIV-infected people who are willing to share and assist newly diagnosed clients during the transition period.
    - Reinforce that an HIV-positive test

means that the client is infected, but does not necessarily mean that the client has AIDS.
  - Arrange for client to see a care provider who is knowledgeable about HIV infection and AIDS.

Assessment

Early intervention after detection of HIV infection can promote health and limit and/or delay disability. A baseline assessment is extremely important at this point. The baseline helps to determine the status of the infection and can help to establish the client's individual norms. Nursing interventions will be based on and tailored to client needs discovered during the assessment. (See Introduction for overview of initial medical assessment.) The nursing assessment in HIV disease should focus on the early detection of constitutional symptoms, opportunistic diseases, and psychosocial problems.

Nursing Assessment for the HIV-Infected Client

Assessment Interventions	Rationales
History Risk factors associated with HIV infection	See Risk Assessment Interview in Primary Prevention section

Assessment Interventions	Rationales	Assessment Interventions	Rationales
Route of infection, estimated date of infection	Clients infected through transfusions tend to progress more rapidly; clients infected through sharing drug injection equipment are at risk of drug-related immune suppression; length of time since infection may give input on immune status	Nutritional assessment	Establishes state of nutritional health; provides opportunity to initiate nutrition education; because weight loss and malnutrition are significantly related to immune function and quality and quantity of life in HIV infection, early intervention is a high priority
History of hepatitis (A, B, or C), other STDs, tuberculosis, frequent viral or parasitic infections, childhood illnesses, cancer	May resurface when immune system becomes compromised; establishes need to educate client about symptoms to report	Medication review: current drug use (prescription, over-the-counter, street) and allergies	Provides information base for interventions related to immune suppressive drugs and drug interactions; alerts providers to continuing treatment issues related to other health problems; provides opportunity to initiate education; decreases risk of allergic reactions
Medical history of acute or chronic diseases, surgeries, transplants, pregnancy	Alerts providers to problems that may be exacerbated by HIV		
Immunization history	Assesses protection status for specific organisms; provides opportunity to encourage needed vaccinations	Previous medical history that may have been an unrecognized early symptom of HIV (i.e., thrush, shingles, etc.)	Helps to determine immune status and length of infection

Assessment Interventions	Rationales	Assessment Interventions	Rationales
Psychosocial history: alcohol/drug/ tobacco use, support systems, career/job, financial state, stress factors, psychiatric disorders, previous losses, coping strategies, self-concept, perception of illness, exercise patterns	Assesses additional stressors on immune system; provides opportunity to initiate appropriate interventions and to encourage interventions to improve immune health	Nose and sinuses: pain, discharge, nosebleeds, obstruction	
Client perception of health status in the following areas: General: chronic fatigue, malaise, low-grade fevers, night sweats, unexplained weight loss, pain	Identified problems may be related to HIV or other health disorders; remember: HIV-infected people can have other acute or chronic health conditions; establishes baseline; provides opportunity for differential diagnosis, initiation of treatment, and education to improve overall health status; establishes need to educate client about signs and symptoms that are important to report; helps to discuss health promotion and disease prevention measures	Respiratory: cough, shortness of breath, chest pain, wheezing, "cold" symptoms	
Head and neck: headaches, stiff neck		Skin: rashes, lesions, blisters, nonhealing wounds, color changes, itching, dryness, changes in hair or nails	
Mouth and throat: lesions on lips, mouth, tongue, throat; pain; sensitivity to acidic, salty, or spicy foods; problems with teeth and gums; difficulty swallowing; bleeding gums; changes in taste		Cardiovascular: chest pain, palpitations, edema, hypertension, hypotension	
		Gastrointestinal: anorexia, nausea, vomiting, changes in bowel habits, persistent diarrhea; rectal pain, itching, lesions, bleeding or ulcerations; retrosternal pain; abdominal pain or cramping; weight loss	
Eyes: blurred vision, photophobia, loss of vision, diplopia		Neurologic: confusion, changes in mental status, memory loss, tremors, personality changes, paresthesia, hypersensitivity in feet, attention deficit, forgetfulness, seizures, syncope	
Ears: decreased hearing acuity, infections, tinnitus			

Assessment Interventions	Rationales
Musculoskeletal: muscle weakness, difficulty walking, arthralgia, myalgia	
Genitourinary: lesions on genitalia (internal or external), itching or burning in vagina, painful sexual intercourse, painful urination, decreased urine output, changes in menstruation, vaginal or penile discharge, impotence, inability to achieve orgasm	
Emotional: indications of anxiety, anger, guilt, frustration, despair, depression, suicidal ideation	
Physical assessment, systems review in the following areas:	
General: vital signs, weight, general appearance, affect, demeanor, muscle tone, hygiene	Signs of advancing HIV disease include fatigue, weakness, neurological changes, depression
Assess for hyperthermia, flushing, diaphoresis	Elevated temperature indicates systemic infection that may be caused by organisms other than HIV

Assessment Interventions	Rationales
Eyes: presence of exudate, inflammation, retinal lesions, hemorrhage, papilledema; check visual acuity	Potential eye problems include conjunctivitis, KS lesions, herpes infection, CMV retinitis, cotton wool spots on retina
Ears: presence of redness, swelling, exudate, lesions, impaired hearing, tinnitus, hygiene	Ear infections and cancers have been noted; hearing problems may be first sign of neuro-cognitive deficit; hearing loss is a quality of life issue that can be treated
Mouth and throat: presence of a variety of mouth lesions including blisters, white-gray patches, painless white lesions on lateral aspect of the tongue, exudate, discolorations, gingivitis, tooth decay or loosening; redness, white patchy lesions, swollen tonsils or exudate in throat; oral hygiene	Mouth is a common site of HIV pathology that may occur early in infection; observe for candidiasis, herpes simplex, KS, oral hairy leukoplakia, aphthous ulcers, gingivitis, periodontitis; throat may reveal candida lesions or inflamed tonsils

Assessment Interventions	Rationales	Assessment Interventions	Rationales
Integumentary system: observe integrity and turgor, general appearance and presence of lesions, eruptions, discoloration, bruises, cyanosis, dryness, delayed wound healing, alopecia	Rashes, bruises, and lesions provide information about general health status; lesions may be caused by herpes zoster, herpes simplex, KS, seborrhea, psoriasis, candida, ringworm, parasites, tinea, molluscum, bacillary angiomatosis; skin may also show signs of drug and allergic reactions, as well as injection sites (track marks)	Abdominal: tenderness, masses, enlarged spleen/liver, hyper- or hypoactive bowel sounds	Identifies problems related to organ enlargement, tumors, chronic drug/alcohol use, pelvic inflammatory disease (PID) and gastrointestinal problems such as cryptosporidiosis, CMV, MAC, isosporiasis, salmonellosis, KS, lymphoma
Cardiovascular: heart rate and rhythm, blood pressure, peripheral edema	Establishes baseline and identifies pre-existing problems	Genitourinary/ Anal: presence of lesions, inflammation or discharge, signs of parasites; women: pelvic exam with Pap smear and specimens for exudate as needed; men: testicular and prostate exams, specimens for exudate as needed	Helps to detect STDs including syphilis, gonorrhea, chlamydia, genital warts, genital herpes; detects genital/rectal cancers, genital/ rectal trauma
Lymph nodes: inspect and palpate; observe for swelling, heat, pain	Detects generalized lymphadenopathy, lymphoma, localized infection		
Respiratory: check rate and depth, presence of rales, dyspnea, cough (may be productive or nonproductive), wheezing, tachypnea, intercostal retractions, dullness on percussion	Opportunistic diseases such as KS, bacterial infections, PCP, histoplasmosis, tuberculosis, coccidioidomycosis, herpes simplex, and cryptococcosis frequently affect pulmonary system	Neurologic: observe for aphasia, ataxia, lack of coordination, sensory loss, tremors, paresthesia, slurred speech, memory loss, apathy, agitation, social withdrawal, pain, vertigo, abnormal reflexes, nuchal rigidity, inappropriate behavior, hemiparesis, decreasing levels of consciousness, depression, seizures, paralysis, coma	Raises level of suspicion for CNS and/or peripheral nervous system pathology common in HIV infection, including toxoplasmosis, PML, cryptococcal meningitis, CNS lymphoma, dementia, encephalitis, demyelinating polyneuropathy; symptoms may also be related to emotional problems and stress

Specific Nursing Diagnoses and Interventions

Altered Health Maintenance

A state in which the HIV-infected individual is unable to identify, manage, and/or seek help to maintain health.

*Author's Note:

Maintenance and/or improvement of immune health may make a difference in long-term morbidity and mortality. Early attention to health promotion is a more productive health tactic than trying to treat an acute exacerbation of disease. The client should be taught about clinical manifestations that may indicate progression of the disease so that prompt medical care can be initiated. The client should be provided with as much information as needed to make health care decisions that will direct nursing and medical intervention.

Related to:

Shock at diagnosis; lack of experience with healthcare or social services; lack of information; lack of motivation; ineffective coping mechanisms (anxiety, depression, denial, avoidance); financial constraints; lack of access to services; religious or cultural beliefs; shame; guilt; fear; desire to hide diagnosis from others

Defining Characteristics:

Unable to initiate entry into health care system

- **Subjective Findings:** Denies that health care is needed ("I feel fine," "I don't have a need to see anyone."); discusses confusion about alternatives and resources; verbalizes frustration with health care system and/or providers

- **Objective Findings:** Apathetic; lack of follow-up to referrals; "no show" for appointments; signs of stress

Outcome Criteria:

Accesses healthcare

Interventions	Rationales
Explain the importance of developing a health care team that is controlled by the client: discuss types of health care currently used; encourage client to develop a relationship with a care provider who will provide long-term medical care and a case manager who will help coordinate services; explore client's desires to use complementary therapies; assist client to develop a comprehensive team that will deal with all aspects of needed care	Empowers the client to take responsibility for care and make critical decisions; reminder that there are needs for physical, dental, emotional, financial, nutritional, and educational support; encourages client to demand interaction of all care providers; supports desire to use non-Western care

Interventions	Rationales
Provide referrals to wide variety of care providers, as requested; use case management as much as possible to decrease complexity of care	Assists client in initiation of care; provides helpful resources
Assure confidentiality	Fear of disclosures about HIV status inhibits many newly diagnosed individuals, keeps them away from care, and/or prevents the development of a care team
Teach signs and symptoms of HIV disease progression, opportunistic disease and somatic problems that need to be reported immediately to health care providers: unexplained weight loss, night sweats, persistent diarrhea, persistent fever, swollen lymph nodes, oral hairy leukoplakia, oral candidiasis, persistent vaginal yeast infections, shortness of breath, persistent cough, headaches, visual changes, changes in digestion, difficulty swallowing, extreme fatigue, numbness in arms/legs, unusual bleeding; pain	Many problems associated with HIV can be controlled if recognized at an early stage; encourages client to develop interactive relationship with care providers

Interventions	Rationales
Initiate discussions about options in combination drug therapy (see Introduction); assess client understanding about ART, desire to initiate therapy, and ability to adhere to complex drug regimens	Starts the process of education about drug therapy; initiates discussion that will assist client to make decisions; provides overview of treatment choices; acknowledges client's right to make decisions and control therapy

Evaluation:

The client:

1. Develops a health care team
2. Lists signs and symptoms that need to be reported
3. Begins process of learning about treatment options

Health Seeking Behaviors

A state in which the HIV-infected client actively seeks ways to alter personal health habits in order to improve function, maintain health, prevent complications, or move to a higher level of wellness.

*Author's Note:

HIV disease progression may be delayed through the promotion of immune health. Also see information related to Primary Prevention.

Related to:

Discovery of HIV status; recognition of current or potential health problems that are related to personal habits; desire to live a productive life despite HIV diagnosis

Defining Characteristics:

Actively explores options

- **Subjective Findings:** Expresses desire to gain control over health status or to seek a higher level of wellness

- **Objective Findings:** Seeks information about health promotion activities; lacks knowledge/skill/support to initiate change

Outcome Criteria:

Develops health promoting behaviors

Interventions	Rationales
Provide verbal and written information on immune health enhancement; areas of specific concern are:	Many newly diagnosed clients are motivated to change detrimental health habits; information provides assistance in determining problem areas

Interventions	Rationales
Nutrition. Institute measures that maintain lean body mass, increase weight, assure appropriate levels of vitamins and micro-nutrients; discourage fad diets and megadosing with vitamins and minerals (10 or more times the Recommended Daily Allowance [RDA]), encourage balanced diet with multivitamin and mineral supplements at 1-2 times the RDA levels; teach ways to prevent food-related illnesses, including using only pasteurized diary products, checking for expiration dates, thoroughly cooking meats and eggs, thawing frozen foods in the refrigerator, washing fresh fruits and vegetables thoroughly, using a separate cutting board for uncooked meats, washing hands before working with food; consult dietitian as needed	Malnutrition can lead to immune suppression; eating contaminated foods can lead to opportunistic infection; proteins and micro-nutrients are needed for immune function and healing; wasting is a major problem for HIV-infected clients at later stages of disease, instituting nutritional changes early may lead to a positive difference in long-term outcome

Interventions	Rationales	Interventions	Rationales
Substance use, including tobacco, alcohol, and drug use. Encourage cessation or moderation of use of all substances that can cause immune system deterioration; refer to cessation education and treatment programs; encourage smokers who do not quit to increase intake of vitamin C to 2-3 grams per day	Any additional immune system suppression can cause serious consequences as disease progresses	*Exercise.* Encourage development of routine exercise program	Assists in the maintenance of lean body mass; stimulates appetite; reduces stress; promotes general health and body function
Skin care. Encourage daily showers, mild soap, use of creams and lotions applied to still-wet skin, and frequent hand washing	Removes organisms on skin that could be transferred to other body parts where opportunistic infections can develop; prevents dry, peeling, cracking skin that is painful and that provides a portal of entry for pathogenic organism	*Stress Management and Relaxation.* Encourage any form of stress reduction or relaxation method that is acceptable to client (see Anxiety and Fear, below)	Stress adversely affects immune function, increasing the risk for disease progression and opportunistic disease; stress can negatively affect nutritional intake, social relationships, and coping ability; adequate rest is required to enhance immune system and replenish energy
Mouth Care. Encourage tooth brushing with a soft brush at least twice a day, flossing at least once a day, good gum care, and dental visits every three months	Helps prevent gum disease and the development of infections with oral pathogens; allows early recognition of oral pathology that, if left untreated, may lead to substantial problems related to pain and poor nutrition	*Exposure to pathogens.* Encourage client to use good housekeeping practices; avoid crowds and "sick" people; wear gloves and a mask when cleaning litter boxes or animal droppings; use barriers to prevent exposure to other STDs during sexual activity	Frequent exposure to new pathogens places strain on the immune system
		Help client assess problematic personal behaviors that negatively affect the immune system	Self-assessment personalizes known problems for the client

Interventions	Rationales	Interventions	Rationales
Assess client for change of lifestyle with the following questions: Is the client motivated to make major and multiple changes in lifestyle? Can client handle only a few problems at a time?	Acknowledges differences in client personalities, abilities, and motivations; HIV may be a major motivator for some clients, for others, it is a stressor that decreases the ability to make changes	If client needs to focus on limited change, assist client to determine 1-2 problems that he or she is willing to work on (client selects problems according to personal abilities, desire for change in the area, and expectations for success); develop strategy and assist with referrals to professionals who work in the areas of nutrition, drug treatment, smoking cessation, stress management, behavior modification, or exercise	Limiting lifestyle changes to a few problem areas that are worked on over time has a better chance in resulting in real behavior change; attempting to change everything at once may be overwhelming for these clients
If client wants to make major changes, determine areas of desired change; develop strategies and assist with referrals to professionals who work in the areas of nutrition, drug treatment, smoking cessation, stress management, behavior modification, relaxation, and exercise	Highly motivated clients will want to see rapid and significant change in their personal health routines; motivation to make major changes in lifestyle has prompted some individuals with other diseases (such as heart disease) to make significant changes in health behaviors		

Interventions	Rationales	Interventions	Rationales
If selected problem is one in which the client wishes to stop an unhealthy behavior (i.e., stop smoking): refer to specialists and/or treatment programs; help client analyze the behavior according to how often it occurs, when it occurs, "triggers" that initiate the behavior, intrinsic rewards of the behavior; assist client to identify manageable steps toward change that can be accomplished within set time limits; explore potential barriers to change and assist with developing plans to overcome barriers; provide praise and rewards as steps in the process are accomplished; use Transtheoretical Model (see Introduction)	Encourages client to assess, plan, and implement change process in a reasoned manner that improves the chance of success; teaches a method of behavior change that can be used in the future for other identified problems; empowers client to stop unhealthy behaviors	If selected problem is one in which the client wishes to *start* a healthy habit (i.e., start an exercise program or initiate ART): provide client with information and resources to explore the behavior; help client develop necessary skills; assist client in developing a program in which the behavior is gradually integrated into daily schedule; promote flexibility that allows for relapse and re-initiation; help to explore potential barriers to success; problem solve to overcome barriers; praise and reward success; use Transtheoretical Model (see Introduction)	Encourages gradual acquisition of health habits; assures continuation of behavior; rewards success but does not punish relapse; assures client that there is support for efforts to improve health status

Evaluation:

The client:

1. Verbalizes an understanding of various health promotion behaviors that can improve immune function
2. Verbalizes intent to develop health promoting behaviors
3. Describes and/or demonstrates health promoting behaviors

Noncompliance (Nonadherence)

A state in which the HIV-infected client desires to adhere to health care requirements but is unable to do so.

*Author's Note

This diagnosis does not apply to the individual who *chooses not to comply* with recommendations of health care providers. Remember that the initial diagnosis of HIV and the demands of the health care system can be overwhelming. Much of the care for HIV infection at this point is focused on monitoring the immune system, providing education, initiating ART, and encouraging health promoting behavior changes. Clients generally feel healthy and may not want to be bothered with frequent reminders of their infection.

Related to:

Desire to hide diagnosis; frequency of clinic visits; long-term nature of the disease requiring prolonged therapy; costs of care; lack of support (from family, peers, employer); knowledge deficit; poor self-esteem; hopelessness; fear; anxiety; distrust of "traditional" health care system; lack of personal interactions with care providers; transportation problems; child care problems; difficulty leaving work for health care appointments; conflicts with personal values, cultural influences, or spiritual beliefs; problems specific to ART including combination drug regimens that are expensive, complicated, require strict adherence, cause side effects, and continue long term

Defining Characteristics:

Inconsistency between expressed desires and actions

- **Subjective Findings:** Discusses difficulties that inhibit adherence; makes statements such as, "I want to do what you say, but I just can't."

- **Objective Findings:** Observations that client is not adhering to recommendations; missed appointments; confusion; progression of disease (development of symptoms, increasing viral loads, decreasing CD4+ T cell counts)

Outcome Criteria:

Decreased barriers to healthcare; behavior changes that demonstrate adherence to treatment and health promotion activities

Interventions	Rationales
Explain procedures and schedules; discuss need for these interventions	Allows client to plan in advance; gives information that is useful if client decides to negotiate ("I can come in for this test, but you'll have to wait until next month for me to see the counselor.")

Interventions	Rationales	Interventions	Rationales
Assess problems and barriers to adherence; discuss ways in which the clinic can assist client with problems such as scheduling late afternoon or evening appointments, combining activities into one visit (blood draws and mental health counseling after physical assessment, for example), considering modification of ART regimen	Identification of problems allows for the development of interventions; assures client that the nurse/clinic will be as flexible as possible to help client meet needs	Recognize that adherence to ART is a multifaceted problem; assess client needs and problems in each of the following areas and initiate interventions that address problems identified for that client:	Assures client that s/he can get assistance in making changes to become more adherent to difficult drug regimens; focuses on individual client need; reinforces the importance of taking ART consistently and correctly in order to prevent or delay problems with drug resistance
Refer to case management, social services, and financial aid to help alleviate problems related to health insurance, money, child care, transportation problems, poor self-esteem, emotional issues, etc.	Adherence is frequently impacted by social and economic issues that may be resolved by accessing appropriate resources		Note: some clients will need special assistance with problems related to child care, substance use, emotional distress, housing, and access to assistance programs; these problems must be addressed in a timely and thorough manner in order to encourage adherence; in some cases, addressing these problems will take precedence over any drug treatment protocols, and decisions may be made to forego ART until those issues are resolved
Implement interventions outlined in Health Seeking Behaviors (above)	Adherence to positive behavior changes are an important aspect of care at this point in HIV infection		

Interventions	Rationales	Interventions	Rationales
Knowledge deficits: assure that the client understands the following: treatment goals and expected benefits of therapy; how the medications work and why adherence is important; what side effects may occur and what to do should they occur; names of prescribed drugs and how to take them (correct dose, frequency of dosing, with or without food, which can be taken together and which cannot be taken together, etc.); discuss information in a quiet and unrushed setting; supplement with written materials that the client can understand (in some cases this will mean translating materials into specific languages, in other cases it may mean providing the information in picture or cartoon formats); as desired by the client, involve supportive significant others in the education process		*Problems with remembering to take drugs:* develop memory aids such as scheduling medications at times when other routine activities occur (brushing teeth, eating breakfast, watching the news, etc.); use divided pill boxes, alarms, beepers, and medication charts; enlist assistance from family, friends, buddy systems, and support groups; simplify the dosing schedule as much as possible *Access problems* (client may not be able to afford drugs, or may lack transportation to pharmacy and clinic for follow-up visits): ask case manager to intervene with state-funded drug assistance programs, locate transportation assistance, explore drug delivery systems (such as by mail) available in many communities	

Interventions	Rationales

Problems with side effects: encourage client to report all problems to care provider; encourage client to continue taking medications until s/he can be seen by the care provider; assure client that modifications can be made in therapy to decrease or eliminate side effect problems

Lack of provider support: maintain open and honest communications with positive reinforcements in an established atmosphere of caring and trust; use a team of providers who maintain frequent contact with client; provide consistent messages to client from all team members; reassure clients that final decisions are always up to them; establish trust by providing acceptance, consistency, respect, individualized care, convenient access to providers, and nonjudgmental attitudes

Evaluation:

The client:

1. Identifies barriers to adherence
2. Verbalizes fears, anxiety, guilt, remorse
3. Develops resources and a plan to increase ability to adhere to recommendations
4. Works within the system to get needs met
5. Uses ART consistently and correctly

Risk for Infection Transmission

A state in which the HIV-infected client is at risk for transmitting HIV to others.

Related to:

Lack of knowledge; sharing of injection equipment; unprotected sexual intercourse; accidents in which others come into contact with client's blood; denial; anger; mental health problems, low self-esteem

Defining Characteristics:

Continuation of risk behaviors

- **Subjective Findings:** Discusses continued risky sexual and injection equipment sharing behaviors; makes statements such as, "They should protect themselves," or "I can't start using condoms because my partner(s) will suspect something is wrong"

- **Objective Findings:** Continuing injection drug use; development of STDs; pregnancy; refuses to disclose status to sex partner(s) or health care providers

Outcome Criteria:

Decreased risk of HIV transmission

Interventions	Rationales	Interventions	Rationales
Initiate related interventions discussed in Primary Prevention: Decisional Conflict, Fear, Powerlessness, Self-Esteem Disturbance, Chronic Low Self-Esteem, Altered Family Processes, Altered Sexuality Patterns, and Ineffective Individual Coping	All are components of risk	Initiate discussion of situations in which the client could potentially place others at risk; ask for specifics about barriers to risk reduction measures, solicit descriptions of successful instances in which risk was eliminated or reduced	Provides information on problems, successes, and willingness to use protection; assesses need for further intervention
Practice Universal Precautions or BSI	HIV-infected people may not know that they are infected or may feel inhibited to disclose their infection status	Identify people who are at risk from this client; assist client to deal with these individuals through disclosing HIV status, negotiating risk reduction methods, requiring consistency in behaviors, family/ couple counseling, and/or severing the relationship	Frequentiy, the people most at risk are those who have long-term sexual or drug using relationships with the client; partners need to be assessed for HIV infection and, if not infected, encouraged to remain uninfected by using risk reduction measures (see Primary Prevention); sometimes the only solution is to sever the relationship (i.e., when client is unwilling to disclose HIV status to peers who share injection equipment)
Teach client about modes of transmission for HIV and risk reduction measures with the following strategies: abstinence, noninsertive sex, use of barrier methods, alternative methods for drug use, not sharing injection equipment, cleaning injection equipment, and disclosure issues (telling health care providers, sexual partners, and drug using peers); require return demonstrations for methods that require the manipulation of equipment	Helps client assess risk and make decisions about activities that place others at risk		

Interventions	Rationales
Assess emotional state, looking for signs that increase transmission risks: anger, desire for revenge, denial, thoughts of suicide, apathy, mental retardation, chronic mental illness, etc.; refer for counseling as needed	Newly diagnosed clients go through an overwhelming amount of emotional stress; reactions are not always consistent with past behaviors or coping mechanisms; negative emotions may take over and influence behaviors
Assess willingness to protect others from infection; unwilling clients need further assistance from public health providers, mental health counselors, support groups, and HIV community-based organizations	This is a difficult ethical issue: nurses are required to maintain client confidentiality but are also expected to protect the health of the community; use all personal and community resources available to help client understand need for taking responsibility to prevent new infections; alternatively, public education helps everyone understand that protection and risk prevention are primarily personal responsibilities

Evaluation:

The client:

1. Lists methods in which HIV can be transmitted
2. Demonstrates activities that decrease the risk of transmission to others
3. Accesses resources for assistance
4. States intent to use risk reduction measures to protect others

Decisional Conflict

A state of indecision between competing choices that involve risk, loss, or challenge to established personal lifestyle or values.

*Author's Note:

Numerous decisions will need to be made by the client at this point, including those related to disclosure of HIV infection, changes in sexual and/or drug using behaviors, changes in plans or goals, development of a health care team, and involvement in various treatment options.

Related to:

Confusing, inconsistent, or incomplete information related to HIV infection; disagreement within support system about best course(s) to take; risks related to the potential loss of relationships, employment, health, personal control; inexperience in decision making; unclear personal value system or a conflict with personal values; ethical dilemmas related to sexuality or drug use; resignation; hopelessness

Defining Characteristics:

Vacillation between choices; delayed decision making

- **Subjective Findings:** Verbalizes uncertainty and negative consequences of perceived alternatives; expresses distress related to diagnosis; discusses frustrations related to health care provider's demands for decisions; denies need to make decisions and/or initiate behavior changes; examines personal values and beliefs

- **Objective Findings:** Physical signs of stress and tension; behaviors that are counter to expressed goals; unrealistic expectations

Outcome Criteria:

Effective, informed decisions

Interventions	Rationales
Assist client to identify the problem, explore options, list positive and negative attributes of each option, identify probable outcomes for each option, and evaluate each option for compatibility with personal values, lifestyle, and support system; reassure client that s/he can make the decision and has the right to do so	Clarifies problem and encourages a thoughtful progression toward a decision that is acceptable to the client; empowers the client to make own decision with support as needed

Interventions	Rationales
If acceptable to the client, encourage involvement of family and significant others in decision making process	Assures others that they remain an important part of the client's life; helps others adopt a supportive position that can prevent future obstructions; gives others the task of providing support for the client
Actively support client's decision even if it is not the decision you would make	Reinforces client's right to make decisions; demonstrates that decisions will not be undermined
If client's decision is illegal or unethical, discuss concerns with the client; seek assistance to resolve professional conflict	HIV can cause a number of ethical conflicts related to balancing the client's right to make decisions and expectations of confidentiality with professional ethics, protecting the health of the community, and upholding the law; these conflicts are complex and require that the nurse explore a variety of avenues for resolution

Evaluation:

The client:

1. States advantages and disadvantages of potential choices
2. Discusses fears and concerns about choices
3. Weighs options and comes to an informed choice
4. States intent to initiate action based on decision
5. Expresses satisfaction with decision(s)

Anxiety

A state in which the client experiences a vague, uneasy feeling in response to a non-specific or unknown threat.

*Author's Note:

Anxiety ranges from mild (a positive state that motivates learning and enhances behavior change efforts), to moderate (in which the individual tends to focus on one issue to the exclusion of others), to panic (in which the client's entire attention is focused on reducing anxiety). The following discussion focuses on moderate anxiety and panic.

Related to:

Diagnosis of HIV; variable course of the disease; unknown response of family or significant others; possibility of rejection; uncertainty

Defining Characteristics:

Stress

- **Subjective Findings:** Makes statements about lack of self-confidence in abilities; verbalizes expectations of the worst possible outcomes; indicates that others are to blame; reports apprehension, worry, nervousness

- **Objective Findings:** Physiologic symptoms of stress, insomnia, fatigue, apprehension; helplessness; nervousness; tension; fear; irritability; anger; withdrawal; lack of initiative; decreased attention span; difficulty learning or remembering; decreased coping ability; avoidance mechanisms

Outcome Criteria:

Anxiety decreased to manageable levels

Interventions	Rationales
Provide reassurance and comfort measures: stay with client, use calm approach, listen attentively, remain silent as appropriate, make no demands on the client, speak slowly and clearly, touch as appropriate (back rub, hand holding, etc.), allow crying, decrease stimulation (provide quiet environment, dim lights)	Initial responses are aimed at decreasing anxiety and apprehension; provides safe, nonthreatening environment
Seek understanding of client's anxiety: ask client to describe situations that initiate anxiety, feelings during episodes of anxiety, fears, and coping efforts	Helps to clarify threat; initiates assessment on which coping strategies can be built; assures client of nurse's concern and desire to help; enhances empathy
Assess for underlying anger: encourage verbalizations about anger; initiate development of appropriate outlets for anger (exercise, involvement in community efforts to prevent spread of HIV, participation in legal action groups, etc.)	Anger is a reasonable reaction to a diagnosis of HIV, but it can become destructive; initiates process to discover causes of anger; suggests appropriate outlets for anger

Interventions	Rationales
Encourage use of relaxation techniques through massage, meditation/ prayer, progressive muscle relaxation, warm baths, guided imagery, biofeedback, music, etc.	Promotes general stress reduction
Refer as needed for mental health counseling, psychiatric interventions, and/or support groups	Intensive therapy and/or medication may be required if anxiety persists or causes problems with ability to function

Evaluation:

The client:

1. Uses effective coping strategy to manage anxiety
2. Verbalizes an increase in comfort levels

Fatigue

A state in which the client feels an overwhelming and sustained sense of exhaustion and decreased ability to maintain usual levels of physical or mental effort; generally not relieved by rest.

*Author's Note:

Fatigue is a common and frustrating symptom of HIV infection. It may occur early in the disease process and may persist over time. Fatigue generally worsens as HIV disease progresses.

Related to:

Infection with HIV; fever; drug use; drug withdrawal; overwhelming emotional demands; depression; stress; insomnia; anemia; malnutrition; drug therapy (ART)

Defining Characteristics:

Overwhelming feeling of tiredness

- **Subjective Findings:** Complains about lack of energy and increasing physical problems; discusses lack of interest in usual relationships/activities; complains about decreased libido; feels guilty about inability to keep up with responsibilities and usual activities

- **Objective Findings:** Inability to maintain usual activities; irritability; decreased ability to concentrate; lethargy; listlessness

Outcome Criteria:

Preservation and efficient use of energy

Interventions	Rationales
Encourage client to verbalize concerns about fatigue: personal meanings, loss of ability to participate in specific activities, effect on emotional state, fears	Acknowledges that fatigue is a real problem, not a result of malingering; initiates assessment of problem

Interventions	Rationales
Help client assess fatigue patterns: ask client to keep a journal of a typical day, making hourly notations about routine activities and energy levels (use a scale of 1 = high energy, 5 = sufficient energy for routine activity, 10 = total exhaustion); analyze diary for times of peak energy, times of exhaustion, and activities associated with each	Assists with development of energy use plan
Assist client to assign priority activities	Provides information on valued daily activities; highlights potentially nonessential activities that can be eliminated
Help client develop schedule that fits priority activities into periods of high energy	Utilizes energy for activities that are important to client
Assure adequate nutritional intake: use high energy supplements as required, cook large meals when energy is high and freeze in single servings for later use	Eating may not be given high priority because of anorexia or apathy; not eating, however, compounds fatigue because energy store is not replenished

Interventions	Rationales
Encourage exercise	Enhances muscle tone, stimulates appetite, increases ability to maintain activity levels, provides distraction, releases endorphins
Help client plan for alternating periods of rest and activity	Replenishes energy stores
Encourage participation in activities that client enjoys, feels are worthwhile, desires to do	Motivation and interest in a worthwhile activity can distract client from feelings of fatigue and/or depression
Determine if fatigue is related to stress or adjustment problems; assist with coping mechanisms; refer for mental health counseling	Depression and anxiety are common responses to a diagnosis of HIV and both can have physical manifestations related to fatigue
Teach energy conservation techniques such as delegation, time management, efficient organization of work spaces, etc.	Decreases energy expenditure while allowing client to remain in control
Encourage use of relaxation techniques such as massage, meditation/prayer, progressive muscle relaxation, warm baths, guided imagery, biofeedback, etc.	Routine daily relaxation increases energy reserves and enhances immune function

Evaluation:

The client:

1. Identifies causes of or contributors to fatigue
2. Discusses frustrations about impact of fatigue on quality of life
3. Establishes priorities for daily activities
4. Develops and follows a schedule that assures a balance of rest and physical activity

Fear

A state in which the client experiences a feeling of dread related to HIV infection and the anticipated chronic disease process.

Related to:

Diagnosis of an incurable infection that causes chronic disease, early death and significant disability; lack of knowledge; negative responses from significant others; unpredictable future

Defining Characteristics:

Feelings of dread or apprehension

- **Subjective Findings:** Describes fearful situations; discusses worries about anticipated losses related to being infected with HIV

- **Objective Findings:** Avoidance behaviors; attention or performance deficits; physical manifestations of fear; social paralysis; anger; grief

Outcome Criteria:

Fear reduced to a manageable level

Interventions	Rationales
Implement interventions described in Anxiety (above)	Fear and anxiety are not the same thing, but many of the clinical manifestations are similar, and nursing interventions can overlap
Encourage client to develop relationships with others who are dealing with similar issues as is acceptable to client: arrange for client to attend support group, enroll in "buddy" programs offered by many HIV service organizations, introduce client to others in clinical setting	Signifies to client that s/he is not alone; allows discussion of specific fears with others who have "been there"; helps client see solutions that may work for him or her
Determine areas of inadequate knowledge or skills and provide appropriate educational experiences	Clarifies misunderstandings and develops skills needed to feel self-reliant and safe

Evaluation:

The client:

1. Identifies personally acceptable coping mechanisms
2. Verbalizes increased levels of comfort

Hopelessness

A state in which the individual sees limited or no alternatives or personal choices available and is unable to mobilize energy on own behalf.

*Author's Note:

HIV is viewed by some as a hopeless situation. At the asymptomatic stage, however, there is the potential for many years of productive life. If hopelessness continues, chances for meaningful existence are reduced. Hope for medical, social, and personal advancements can make the client's remaining life meaningful.

Related to:

Diagnosis of chronic and potentially lethal infection; perceived inability to achieve valued goals (education, career, children); loss or impairment of a valued relationship; stress; loss of spiritual belief system; multiple losses

Defining Characteristics:

Appears to have given up

- **Subjective Findings:** Expresses profound, overwhelming apathy in response to a situation perceived as impossible with no solutions, "I might as well give up now"; feels "empty, drained"; discusses lack of ambition, interest, initiative; verbalizes feelings of vulnerability and helplessness

- **Objective Findings:** Slowed responses; lack of energy; increased or decreased sleep; flat affect; decreased ability to solve problems and make decisions; unable to recognize solutions or sources of hope; anorexia and weight loss; severe depression; social withdrawal; anger; negative thought processes; confusion; poor communication skills; unrealistic perceptions; pessimism; suicidal ideation

Outcome Criteria:

Future focus

Interventions	Rationales	Interventions	Rationales
Encourage verbalizations about situation and lack of options	Motivates client to state inner feelings and get them "out on the table" for future discussion; assesses problem from client's perspective; initiates communication process related to observed resignation; validates feelings; promotes trusting relationship	Encourage enhanced relationships with significant others: promote opportunities for positive interactions; provide supportive counseling as needed; help client accept needed assistance from others	Reinforces the need for close human relationships; reminds client that depression and rejection can result in the loss of important others who are needed now more than ever; gives others a positive support role in client's life at a time when they may be questioning whether they can really help their loved one
Initiate guided life review	Provides client with historical perspective of past successes; reinforces intrinsic worth; reminds client of important personal relationships; demonstrates that the client is more than his or her current HIV diagnosis	Determine client's need to expand spiritual support base, if desired; encourage ties to preferred religious group; if client has no preferred religion, explore various spiritual philosophies that may provide comfort; also see Spiritual Distress (below)	All humans have a spiritual base whether it is formally defined or not; spiritual supports (if desired by the client) can provide comfort in times of stress
Help client identify sources of hope and support (i.e., significant others, realistic goals, spirituality, etc.)	Assesses potential alternatives to feeling of hopelessness; recognizes personal values; encourages client to embrace rather than deny resources	Reinforce hope: recognize client's intrinsic worth; view the client as a whole person, not a disease process; expect client to participate in own care	Promotes self-esteem; reminds client that his or her life should be viewed as an entire process of past, present, and future possibilities; gets client actively involved; mastery over self-care enhances confidence in abilities

Interventions	Rationales
Facilitate realistic goal setting or restructuring of goals: examine current goal structure and determine if any are truly impossible; eliminate goals that are assigned low priority in light of HIV diagnosis; focus on goals that can be accomplished within 5-10 years	Reassesses goals (and life) in light of HIV diagnosis: often clients discover that a goal previously thought to be of highest importance is no longer desired because of revised life priorities; new goals may be developed that are more timely or are directly related to HIV (i.e., becoming active in projects to teach others about HIV infection; developing fund raising projects for AIDS research, etc.)
Support grieving process as former goals are lost (see Anticipatory Grieving, below)	Acknowledges losses related to HIV
Facilitate decision making (see Decisional Conflict above)	The inertia of hopelessness requires some kind of impetus for action; decision making can provide that motivation
Assess need for suicide prevention measures (see Risk for Suicide, below)	Hopelessness may lead to the desire to "end it all"

Interventions	Rationales
Initiate referrals as needed through support groups, mental health counseling, education/ counseling to support goal achievement, religious leaders, etc.	Professional assistance helps client focus on issues and progress toward goal achievement

Evaluation:

The client:

1. Explores positive aspects of life prior to diagnosis (life review)
2. Reconsiders personal life values
3. Reinforces positive relationships with significant others
4. Expresses confidence in ability to deal with immediate issues related to HIV and health care
5. Sets realistic goals
6. Exhibits sufficient energy levels to progress toward goals
7. Demonstrates initiative, self-direction, and autonomy in decision making and follow-up activities

Powerlessness

A state in which the client perceives a lack of personal control in life after a diagnosis of HIV infection.

*Author's Note:

Facilitating empowerment is particularly important because the individual with HIV infection often experiences overwhelming feelings of loss of control.

Related to:

Positive HIV antibody test; lack of knowledge; expectations that HIV causes inevitable, uncontrollable consequences; feelings of doom; control perceived as a highly valued aspect of personal life; history of helplessness, dependence on others as a lifestyle

Defining Characteristics:

Perceived lack of power

- **Subjective Findings:** Expresses discomfort or hostility over inability to control situation; verbalizes feelings of lack of control over outcome; expresses dissatisfaction and frustration; discusses fears related to loss of abilities, control, or self-concept associated with disease

- **Objective Findings:** Develops behaviors and attitudes that indicate dissatisfaction with lack of power such as apathy, aggression, acting-out behaviors, anxiety, depression, resignation, passivity

Outcome Criteria:

Exerts appropriate control

Interventions	Rationales
Encourage client to talk about feelings, perceptions, and fears related to assuming personal responsibility for health care	Initiates assessment of issues that are most important to client

Interventions	Rationales
Discuss consequences of allowing others to control decisions about health and life after HIV diagnosis	Points out that others may not be able to make optimal decisions for the client because only the client knows all of the factors that should be considered in making those decisions
Explain options, answer questions, clarify confusing issues	Information is power: knowing what can be done provides hope and gives data to consider when making decisions
Encourage client to take personal responsibility for health care	Includes aspects of Altered Health Maintenance, Health Seeking Behaviors, Risk for Infection, Decisional Conflict, and Fear (see above)
Help client determine areas where it is safe, comfortable, or feasible to exert more control; assist with development of plan to assume more control in these areas	Enhances frequency of situations where there is a good chance of success

Evaluation:

The client:

1. Identifies control issues that are stressful
2. Realistically assesses factors that can be controlled by self
3. Makes and follows through on decisions

Situational Low Self-Esteem

A state of negative self-evaluation that develops in response to a diagnosis of HIV infection in a person who had a positive self-image prior to diagnosis.

Related to:

Diagnosis of HIV infection; anticipations of relationship problems, loss of relationships, inability to continue education or work goals; negative social or cultural definitions of HIV and AIDS; discrimination based on diagnosis and/or disclosure of participation in risky activities

Defining Characteristics:

Negative changes in self-image due to HIV infection

- **Subjective Findings:** Makes self-negating statements; expresses guilt, worthlessness or shame; evaluates self as incapable, inadequate, or inferior because of HIV status; feels powerless, hopeless, or helpless; expects social discrimination because of HIV status

- **Objective Findings:** Self-negating behaviors; indecisiveness; inability to set goals or make decisions; poor problem-solving skills; signs of depression; self-abusive behaviors (including substance use, sexually acting-out behavior and assuming the role of victim); denial of problems; projecting blame and responsibility to others

Outcome Criteria:

Enhanced self-esteem

Interventions	Rationales
Explore self-perception issues with client: examine negative perceptions, discuss reasons for self-criticism or guilt, identify significance of HIV diagnosis as it influences self-esteem	Provides opportunities for understanding where negative self-image comes from; demonstrates acceptance of client despite HIV diagnosis; reinforces self-worth
Reinforce previous positive self-esteem by exploring client's positive attributes and accomplishments: identify strengths, point out attractive physical features, reinforce past accomplishments	Identifies presence of positive attributes; enhances self-esteem; reminds client that HIV is only a part of personal identity
Recommend activities that show and reinforce personal capabilities: encourage realistic goal setting, increased responsibility, self-evaluation, and social interaction	Expressing confidence in client's ability provides external source of esteem that may become internalized as successes accumulate

Interventions	Rationales
Facilitate client interactions with others who have dealt with a diagnosis of HIV infection by contacting HIV service organizations to determine types of services available (many provide one-on-one encounters, support groups, and educational and volunteer opportunities)	Shows client that s/he is not alone in having to deal with these issues; provides role models who have come through the initial diagnosis with self-esteem and egos intact; provides opportunities for esteem enhancing activities among non-judgmental peers
If problems persist, initiate appropriate referrals to mental health professionals	Situational low self-esteem may progress to chronic low self-esteem if precipitating factor is allowed to become the overriding concern in the client's life

Evaluation:

The client:

1. Discusses self-perceptions
2. Realistically analyzes personal capabilities
3. Reflects on positive personal attributes
4. Reassesses impact of HIV infection on self-evaluation

Altered Family Processes

A state in which a family that normally functions effectively experiences a challenge to its functional status when a family member becomes infected with HIV.

*Author's Note:

Functional families tend to reintegrate after a major stressor and continue to provide support while dysfunctional families, without enormous amounts of assistance, may disintegrate with the occurrence of major stressors. Strong families that remain supportive to the HIV-infected client need assistance to deal with problems that will arise throughout the disease process.

Related to:

Disclosure of diagnosis of HIV infection; realization that there is a potential infection risk for others in the family (i.e., sexual partners and/or children born after infection occurred); behavior changes that are required to decrease risk of infection to other family members (families are often intimately involved in sexual or drug using activities); disruption of family routines; change in role of a family member; breach of trust among members related to discovery of sexual activity or drug use; financial burdens on the family related to health care and potential changes in employment or income; blame; guilt; fear; anger

Defining Characteristics:

Family system does not adapt to changes

- **Subjective Findings:** *Client* reports that family is not being supportive; discusses loss of intimacy with family members and feelings of being outcast; blames self for all familial problems; feels family does not respect, support, or care for him or her; *Family Member*(s) express anger, guilt, shame, rejection

- **Objective Findings:** Poor communication within family; physical, emotional, spiritual, or safety needs of individual not met by family

Outcome Criteria:

Maintenance of supportive family structure

Interventions	Rationales
Encourage family to discuss the issues that have developed: Are there concerns about transmission to other family members? What can be expected as far as disease progression and disability are concerned? What resources are available? etc.	Initiates discussion of difficult issues; identifies knowledge deficits
Teach family members basic information about HIV infection: transmission, protection, stages of disease progression, available treatments, need for family support	Allays anxiety and fear, provides basis for realistic planning
Assess ability of the family to provide needed support: Is client still a welcomed family member? What is the immediate response - rejection or acceptance? What are the strengths of the family unit? Is there a risk that this stressor is too much for the family to manage?	Provides basis for intervention recommendations

Interventions	Rationales
Assist family to resolve conflicts by encouraging expressions of guilt, hostility and anger; refer to family therapy as appropriate	Helps family members identify real issues ("Is it my fault?"; "I love you, but I can't accept the fact that you are gay/use drugs."; "I don't want to watch you die."); facilitates interactions that can lead to positive change; defuses potentially volatile situations
Provide continuing support to individual within family who is infected with HIV	Primary responsibility is to client: sometimes best solution is to help client sever ties with non-supportive family and develop new relationships (at least until family members are better able to accept the client)

Evaluation:

Family members:

1. Verbalize concerns about family function
2. Communicate concerns to other family members
3. Resolve issues
4. Maintain support system for family members

Anticipatory Grieving

A state in which the client and/or significant others experience reactions in response to an expected significant loss.

*Author's Note:

Although the burden of loss usually occurs later in the course of HIV infection, some losses may occur immediately. These can include losses that are not controlled by the client (a partner leaving, getting fired) or those that are controlled by the client (decisions to quit school, not have children, move to a new location). All losses are difficult, even those that are seen as desirable and appropriate by the client.

Related to:

Expectations that HIV infection will progress to disability and death; anticipated losses may include loss of function, capability, income, possessions, independence, relationships, control, body image, self-respect, goal attainment, having children, watching children mature, support systems, spiritual base, or dignity as well as actual death

Defining Characteristics:

Expectations of loss

- **Subjective Findings:** Expresses distress at potential losses; verbalizes concerns about anticipated losses that are personally significant; acknowledges decreased libido; feels resigned to fate, anxious, lonely, tired; blames self for infection

- **Objective Findings:** Denial; anger; bargaining; guilt; sorrow; depression; change in social and communication patterns; withdrawal; tearfulness; ambivalence; sleep and appetite disturbances

Outcome Criteria:

Realistic appraisal of anticipated losses

Interventions	Rationales
Encourage client to identify losses that are anticipated	Assesses extent of anticipatory grief; provides useful information for further interventions
Help client assess each anticipated loss in a realistic manner; ask client to describe personal meanings related to each potential loss; provide information that can help with assessment	Many newly diagnosed clients feel that their lives are over; discussing the spectrum of infection can give the client hope that the anticipated physical losses are not likely to occur for quite some time and that many social, career, education, family, and recreation activities can be continued in the immediate future; decreases anxiety
Facilitate grieving for those losses that are imminent	Acknowledges all losses; validates the importance of each loss; provides the basis for closure and growth

Interventions	Rationales
Encourage client to share concerns with supportive individuals such as family, friends, counselors, religious/spiritual leaders, support group peers, etc.	Reinforces the importance of the support system that will be needed as client advances through the disease process; gives supportive individuals insight into client's problems; assures significant others that they are a valued and needed part of the client's life
Initiate interventions discussed in Decisional Conflict, Anxiety, Fatigue, Fear, Hopelessness, Powerlessness, Altered Family Processes (above)	All of these factors are components of grief and need to be addressed

Evaluation:

The client/significant other:

1. Discusses anticipated losses
2. Realistically assesses losses according to risk of occurrence and timing of occurrence
3. Expresses grief
4. Develops plans for allaying, delaying, or coping with future losses
5. Shares concerns with significant others

Altered Sexuality Patterns

A state in which an individual or partner expresses concerns about the client's sexuality as it is or how it will be affected by HIV.

Related to:

Fear of transmitting or contracting HIV infection; fear of contracting other STDs; fear of rejection if disclosure of infection is made

Defining Characteristics:

Concern over the effect of an HIV diagnosis on sexual function

- **Subjective Findings:** Expresses concern about sexuality; identifies involvement in sexual behaviors that place others at risk for HIV infection; discusses fears about changes in sexual function if risk reducing measures are instituted; verbalizes guilt, shame, or stigma; discusses frustrations related to sexuality; acknowledges change in sexual behavior or activities

- **Objective Findings:** Reluctance to discuss sexual issues; guilt; fear; shame

Outcome Criteria:

Development of safe and satisfactory sexual function

Interventions	Rationales
Implement interventions discussed in Altered Sexuality in Primary Prevention	Primary prevention issues influence risk of transmission to others, sexuality, and ability to change current level of sexual function

Interventions	Rationales	Interventions	Rationales
Get a sexual history	Assesses usual sexual practices; provides basis for discussions related to continuing sexual expression while protecting partner(s); initiates discussion and presents sexuality as an acceptable topic	As possible, involve client's partner in discussions of sexual possibilities (the partner has a vested interest in this discussion): discuss risks related to becoming infected, issues related to enforced celibacy, concerns about pregnancy, developing creative and fulfilling sexual interactions while maintaining safety	Promotes a continuing sexual outlet for both partners; encourages mutual problem solving; assists in maintenance of relationship; focuses on safety
Encourage holistic exploration of personal issues that affect sexual function: What does sexual intercourse mean to the client? Does the use of a condom demean, insult, or create gender issues for the client or the sexual partner? What are the client's cultural, religious, and ethical influences related to sexual function? How does/will the partner respond to sexual activity in light of the HIV diagnosis?	Sexuality is an important aspect of health; it is influenced by a wide variety of factors, any one of which can create potential blocks to healthy sexual activities in the HIV-infected client	Teach spectrum of sexuality and relate to safe, risk reducing, and high-risk behaviors; discuss positive and negative features of sexual options	Assists in evaluation of options for sexual expression in HIV infection
		Provide reassurance and encourage experimentation in alternate forms of sexual expression; provide "practice sessions"; simulate client-partner verbal interactions; practice negotiations in role plays and develop condom use skills with dildos or cucumbers to simulate an erect penis; develop female condom use skills with plastic models of the vagina	Decreases inhibitions that can limit client's willingness to expand choices in sexual expression; decreases anxiety; provides support in a safe environment

Interventions	Rationales
Discuss factors related to HIV infection that may negatively affect sexual function, including fatigue, fear, anxiety, guilt, blame, anger, loss of libido, apathy, stress	Initiates discussions that can lead to problem solving
Use appropriate humor and encourage client and partner to use humor as a way of relieving embarrassment	Acknowledges that sexuality is a sensitive issue; sends message that sexual activity can/should be an enjoyable, fun, healthy experience

Evaluation:

The client:

1. Discusses concerns about sexuality
2. States intent to implement strategies for sexual interactions that decrease/eliminate risk of transmitting HIV
3. Verbalizes satisfaction with sexual function

Ineffective Individual Coping

A state in which an individual experiences an inability to adapt, solve problems, or manage stressors related to a diagnosis of HIV infection because of inadequate resources.

Related to:

Diagnosis of HIV with resultant health care requirements and potential lifestyle changes; disruption of relationships; poverty; inadequate support system; low self-esteem; stress overload; hopelessness; powerlessness; culturally related conflicts with life experiences (especially homosexuality, drug use, sex work)

Defining Characteristics:

Ineffective coping; lack of resource support necessary for coping

- **Subjective Findings:** Verbalizes inability to cope with situations related to HIV infection; worries about inability to meet role expectations; expresses anxiety; reports overwhelming stress; admits to an inability to ask for assistance and fear of becoming dependent

- **Objective Findings:** Difficulty with problem solving and decision making; destructive behavior toward self or others; inability to meet basic needs; low self-esteem; impaired self-efficacy; inability to identify or access resources; low morale; lack of clear, realistic goals; hopelessness; social withdrawal

Outcome Criteria:

Enhanced ability to cope

Interventions	Rationales	Interventions	Rationales
Implement interventions described in Altered Health Maintenance, Health Seeking Behaviors, Decisional Conflict, Anxiety, Fear, Hopelessness, Powerlessness, Situational Low Self-Esteem, Altered Family Processes, and Altered Sexuality Patterns (above)	All of these issues influence coping ability	Ask client to describe previous encounters with stressors; encourage client to critique encounters to discover helpful and less helpful coping strategies	Allows reflection; encourages development of new coping methods that can be applied to future confrontations; reinforces assurance that positive coping can occur
Explore variety of methods to enhance coping ability including anger control, anxiety reduction, confusion management, counseling, crisis intervention, distraction, environmental management, emotional support, meditation, progressive muscle relaxation, reminiscence therapy, substance use treatment, support groups, group therapy, activity therapy, art therapy, biofeedback, family therapy, hypnosis, etc.	Informs client of a number of alternatives to help develop coping strategies	Help client identify stressors that cannot be dealt with directly; explore stress reducing practices that help with generalized stress reduction such as exercise, yoga, meditation, relaxation techniques	Reinforces ability to care for self despite lack of power in specific areas
		Enhance coping skills: work through a problem-solving exercise on one of the client's identified problem areas; help client develop plan; encourage implementation of the plan; evaluate effectiveness of plan and assist with necessary modifications; recognize and praise successes	Models problem-solving behaviors; provides opportunity for success; encourages generalization of problem-solving process to other problem areas

Interventions	Rationales
Refer to support groups, counselors, or others who have an understanding of the client's situational stressors	Provides a network of knowledgeable individuals who can provide situation-specific support and guidance

Evaluation:

The client:

1. Discusses issues that appear to be overwhelming
2. Acknowledges personal strengths and uses those strengths to plan coping strategies
3. Accepts support from nursing relationship and other resources
4. Develops coping plan and follows through with appropriate actions

Ineffective Denial

A state in which an individual consciously or unconsciously attempts to disavow a diagnosis of HIV infection in order to reduce anxiety or fear.

*Author's Note:

Denial can result in a detrimental effect on personal health and create a risk for transmission of HIV to others. Refusing to let HIV dominate one's life, however, is not ineffective denial. It is, instead, a healthy way to cope with a difficult diagnosis. The following discussion focuses on denial that causes or could potentially cause detrimental health outcomes.

Related to:

Inability to acknowledge risk of being infected with HIV, accuracy of HIV test, or possibility of HIV diagnosis; lack of symptoms in early infection; knowledge deficit; low self-esteem; feelings of inadequacy, guilt, loneliness, despair, failure, anger, frustration, anxiety

Defining Characteristics:

Inability to accept diagnosis of HIV infection

- **Subjective Findings:** States that symptoms are related to other causes such as a cold, the flu, stress, PMS, not enough sleep, etc.; makes statements such as, "I feel fine, I can't have HIV."; "People with AIDS look awful and feel worse."; feels anxious; accepts diagnosis but denies personal implications of the diagnosis

- **Objective Findings:** Refuses to seek health care; does not perceive dangers inherent in denial (for self or others); uses home remedies to treat early symptoms; minimizes symptoms; refuses to discuss plans for children who may need physical and emotional support as a result of parent's infection

Outcome Criteria:

Acknowledges HIV infection

Interventions	Rationales	Interventions	Rationales
Assess effect of denial on client's health and risk to others: if risk is acceptable, continue therapeutic health care relationship without forcing the denial issue; if not acceptable, continue with following suggestions for interventions	If there are no symptoms and the disease is not progressing aggressively, delaying treatment does not cause major concern; if client is posing no risk to others (i.e., is celibate, engages only in safe sexual activities, or does not share injection equipment), the public health issue is eliminated	Explore client's interpretation of the situation in the following areas: why the test came back positive, history of risk, explanation of symptoms, knowledge of HIV versus other diseases with similar symptoms; fears and anxieties	Assesses knowledge base; provides input for planning future interventions; supports therapeutic relationship
Determine basis for denial	Provides important assessment information that may lead to focused interventions such as those described in Noncompliance (Nonadherence), Decisional Conflict, Anxiety, Fear, Hopelessness, Powerlessness, Situational Low Self-Esteem, Altered Family Processes, and Altered Sexuality Patterns (above); also see Self-Esteem Disturbance and Chronic Low Self-Esteem in Primary Prevention	Use a focus of protecting the client to initiate risk reduction discussions	Encourages client to learn and use safe or risk reducing behaviors that will protect others in the community; see Primary Prevention
		Correct inaccuracies and deficiencies in knowledge base	Clarifies information and limits ability to use erroneous information as basis for denial
Avoid direct confrontation of denial	Reduces risk of entrenching denial; prevents destruction of therapeutic relationship		

Evaluation:

The client:

1. Identifies fears and anxieties related to a diagnosis of HIV infection
2. Protects others from exposure to HIV
3. Develops a knowledge base that supports acceptance of infection
4. Implements alternative coping strategies
5. Experiences reduction in fear and/or anxiety

Risk for Violence, Self-Directed

A state in which an individual is at high risk of killing him or herself.

*Author's Note:

For some individuals, the initial diagnosis of HIV infection causes such severe stress that it can lead to suicidal ideation, suicide attempt, and successful suicide—a desire for ultimate control over life.

Related to:

Pervasively negative connotations of the general public related to HIV infection and AIDS; expectations of stigmatization and discrimination related to diagnosis; perceived inability to deal with disability and pain; lack of a cure; knowledge deficit related to course of HIV disease and treatment options; depression; ineffective coping skills; lack of support system; desire for ultimate control over life

Defining Characteristics:

Death seen as the best solution

- **Subjective Findings:** Expresses desire to die; makes frequent statements such as "I should end it all," "My family would be better off if I were dead," or "I can't live with this hanging over my head."

- **Objective Findings:** History of suicidal ideation or suicide attempt, especially as a means to deal with life problems; depression; low self-esteem; hopelessness; helplessness; powerlessness; escalating substance use

Outcome Criteria:

Suicide attempt prevented

Interventions	Rationales
Demonstrate concern about client's welfare	HIV-infected clients may feel that no one really cares; the nurse has an opportunity to provide assurances of human caring
Determine if client has specific suicide plan, history of self-abuse or suicide attempt, access to lethal weapons or medications, or has recently expressed some relief from a depressive episode	Indicates high level of risk
Provide immediate intervention if client is judged to be at high risk: may include anything from constant observation by significant other to a session with a mental health professional to hospitalization	Primary focus is to prevent suicide attempt
Ask client to make a verbal nonsuicide contract that is time limited: "Can you promise me that you won't do anything until after our appointment tomorrow?"	Buys time; provides experience with self-control; allows chance for continuing intervention

Interventions	Rationales
Refer for mental health counseling	Interactions with professionals can help client understand problems and develop alternative coping mechanisms
After immediate risk has passed, initiate care plan that will decrease risk of future suicide attempts; implement interventions described in Altered Health Maintenance, Health Seeking Behaviors, Non-compliance (Nonadherence), Decisional Conflict, Anxiety, Fatigue, Fear, Hopelessness, Powerlessness, Situational Low Self-Esteem, Altered Family Processes, Altered Sexuality Patterns, and Ineffective Individual Coping (above)	All are potentially related to client's desire to die

Evaluation:

The client:

1. Verbalizes intent to continue living
2. Accepts assistance from variety of resources
3. Develops effective alternative coping strategies

Spiritual Distress

A state of disruption in the individual's belief or value system that provides strength, hope, and meaning to life and that transcends the individual's biological and psychosocial nature.

*Author's Note:

Many feel that this is such a personal area that nurses should not get involved. If a need is assessed, however, it is appropriate to spend time helping the client deal with spiritual issues as long as the nurse's personal beliefs are not forced onto the client. Remember that individuals who are facing long-term illness, disability, pain, and death have a heightened awareness of their need for support from a higher power. Spirituality includes more than a relationship with a higher power, however. Additional components include personal satisfaction, meaning and purpose in life, caring and relatedness to others, forgiveness, growth, and a journey toward a feeling of completeness.

Related to:

Diagnosis of HIV infection; real or anticipated losses related to diagnosis; feelings that spiritual system has failed; lack of previously developed spiritual values; denial of need for spirituality; separation from religious, cultural, or family ties

Defining Characteristics:

Searching for a spiritual base

- **Subjective Findings:** Questions belief system, relationship with higher power, personal significance, purpose of suffering; feels infection is incongruent with previously held beliefs; expresses ambivalence about beliefs; describes a sense of spiritual emptiness; initiates discussions about meaning of life, death, disease; relates history of negative response from religious leader(s) or congregation(s); expresses anger toward God; describes HIV as a punishment for previous behaviors; blames self or denies responsibility

- **Objective Findings:** Requests spiritual assistance; appetite and sleep disturbances; crying

Outcome Criteria:

Receives spiritual support and comfort

Interventions	Rationales
Communicate nonjudgmental acceptance of wide variety of spiritual beliefs and practices; defend client's right to develop own spirituality even if it doesn't match yours or conform to social norms; be especially sensitive to cultural facets of spirituality	Encourages client to discuss spiritual issues; promotes empathy and understanding
Assess need for spiritual interventions based on defining characteristics (above)	Client comments and demeanor are helpful cues for initiating spiritual supports

Interventions	Rationales
If a need is determined, provide opportunities to discuss issues: focus on helping the client verbalize concerns rather than solving the problems; support any spiritual activity that does not compromise client's health; be nonjudgmental and set aside own spiritual beliefs in order to support client's spiritual development	Encourages "thinking out loud" that can help in values clarification; conveys concern for the entire client, not just HIV; allows expression of negative feelings; enhances values clarification
Refer, as requested by the client, to spiritual or religious leaders or counselors	Professional assistance can help client establish meaningful relationships with higher power, self, and others; promotes self-acceptance, hope and a sense of purpose

Evaluation:

The client:

1. Continues and enhances positive spiritual practices
2. Explores options for spiritual development and support
3. Expresses satisfaction with belief system and associated supports
4. Experiences enhanced inner peace and decreased somatic and emotional distress

Chapter V

Tertiary Prevention

As HIV disease progresses, the immune system becomes less able to protect the client from pathogens and cancers. Specific symptoms and opportunistic diseases that will move the client into a formal diagnosis of AIDS may develop (see Introduction). Nursing care becomes more complicated as the client's immune system deteriorates and new problems develop. The goals of caring for symptomatic HIV-infected clients are to:

1. Establish & maintain effective antiretroviral therapy (ART).
2. Manage problems caused by HIV infection and its treatment.
3. Maximize quality of life.
4. Promote adjustment to a chronic disease and its acute exacerbations.
5. Prevent and/or treat opportunistic infections.
6. Prevent further transmissions.

Symptomatic HIV disease manifests itself in a number of ways. Symptoms range from irritating and painful (skin rashes or mouth sores) to potentially lethal (pneumonia or lymphoma). Symptoms may be persistent over several months or years or may recur intermittently. As the immune system deteriorates, the symptoms become more difficult to treat and are more likely to disturb normal life activities.

Recent advances in the development of antiretroviral drugs and research that confirms the benefits of multidrug therapy have changed the focus of care for HIV-infected clients, especially at the tertiary stage. Although some clients will continue to refuse ART and others will be unable to tolerate the side effects and still others will have social and economic reasons to forego therapy, the major thrust of medical care at this time lies in the use of pharmacologic interventions. ART has afforded continued health and prolonged life to many HIV-infected people, and its efficacy has brought hope to an epidemic that was for so long without hope. Because of this, many clinicians will encourage ART for all HIV-infected clients at this stage of their disease. Major concerns for nursing care related to ART will continue to focus on client education, encouragement, communication, and support regardless of the decisions made about ART.

Nursing care at the tertiary stage can take place in a number of locations, depending on the nature and severity of the symptoms and on the client's choices for health care. Many problems can continue to be taken care of on an out-patient basis with or without home care. During acute exacerbations of symptoms and opportunistic diseases, care may be provided through hospital medical/surgical, emergency, or intensive care areas. In some cases, care may be provided by long-term care facilities or hospice providers, although this is generally not needed until the terminal phases of the disease.

Assessment

Nursing assessment is a continuing need because early recognition and treatment of opportunistic diseases and somatic problems can be life saving. Having a baseline assessment will help the nurse recognize changes in usual functional levels (see Secondary Prevention). A thorough systems review is needed because of the interactive nature of problems related to HIV infection. It will, of course, be important to focus on problem areas identified through the history and physical exam.

Nurses must also continue to assess psychosocial parameters. Quality-of-life issues become especially important at this point: family support, economic stability, feelings of self-worth and social interactions are all important components of quality of life.

It is important to assess the client's personal desires; this will give the nurse information that can be used to help the client maintain an acceptable standard of life. Acceptable quality of life changes during the course of HIV disease, so expect to reassess this issue on a regular basis.

Specific Nursing Diagnoses and Interventions

Health Seeking Behaviors

A state in which the HIV-infected client actively seeks ways to alter personal health habits in order to improve function, maintain health, prevent complications, or move to a higher level of wellness.

*Author's Note:

At the tertiary stage, there may be an enhanced desire for health promoting activities, stimulated by the development of uncomfortable symptoms. For some clients, activities initiated during the asymptomatic phase will be continued. For others, however, symptom development will provide the first stimulus to try to improve health status. In other cases, symptom development causes a fatalistic outlook and previous health activities may be abandoned (i.e., resuming smoking).

Related to:

Development of symptoms; recognition of current or potential health problems that are related to personal habits; desire to prevent or relieve symptoms or opportunistic diseases

Defining Characteristics:

Seeks information about health promotion activities

- **Subjective Findings:** Expresses desire to gain control over health status or to seek a higher level of wellness; requests support in exploring options

- **Objective Findings:** Lacks knowledge, skill, or support to initiate change; seeks resources

Outcome Criteria:

Continues or initiates health promoting behaviors

Interventions	Rationales
Provide verbal and written information on immune health enhancement; see Health Seeking Behaviors in Secondary Prevention for information about basic interventions; additional measures include the following:	As symptoms develop, the desire to maintain health increases
ART. Provide appropriate information to allow informed decisions; see Noncompliance (Nonadherence) in Secondary Prevention for details about helping clients use multidrug therapy	To date, ART has provided the most effective therapy against HIV

Interventions	Rationales	Interventions	Rationales
Nutrition. If client is underweight, encourage the addition of 20-30 pounds; encourage high-calorie, high-protein diet; encourage 6 meals per day	An acute episode of one of the opportunistic infections can cause rapid weight loss; having a 20-30 pound "cushion" provides some protection for borderline clients who can end up 10-20% below ideal weight during one of these episodes	*Exercise.* Encourage a routine exercise program as tolerated by the client; develop an exercise regimen that increasingly enhances strength and stamina	Helps in the utilization of energy; promotes feelings of physical well being; contributes to self-sufficiency
Substance use, including tobacco, alcohol, and street drug use. Continue to encourage cessation or moderation of all of these substances	In addition to immune system suppression, these substances can cause nutritional problems and damage to a variety of organs including the lungs, liver, GI tract, and cardiovascular system	*Stress-Management/ Relaxation.* Continue to encourage stress reduction and relaxation methods	Assists client to conserve energy, focus on primary concerns, and deal with the stresses of chronic disease
Skin care. In addition to good skin care, encourage daily assessment of the skin for new lesions and/or changes in existing lesions	Identifies developing problems; encourages client to take an active role in health care	*Exposure to pathogens.* Remind client of measures to prevent coming into contact with potentially dangerous organisms by avoiding crowds and people with communicable disease	Exposure to new pathogens can lead to acute illnesses
Mouth Care. Continue to encourage careful mouth care	Oral health is needed to maintain proper nutritional intake; oral manifestations of HIV are frequently painful and distracting	Help client assess areas of need, develop plans and initiate interventions to make positive changes that improve health status	See Health Seeking Behaviors in Secondary Prevention

Evaluation:

The client:

1. Verbalizes an understanding of various health promotion behaviors that can improve immune function
2. Verbalizes intent to develop health promoting behaviors
3. Describes and/or demonstrates health promoting behaviors

Ineffective Management of Therapeutic Regimen

A state in which the HIV-infected client experiences difficulty integrating treatments into his/her daily life.

*Author's Note:

The treatment of HIV infection in the tertiary stage can require complex and confusing medication regimens. Clients often complain about having to take 10 or more pills a day on different and specific time schedules. This is compounded by medical requirements for laboratory work, frequent physician visits, inhalation or physical therapies, management of appliances for infusion therapy, and other common requirements for treatment of HIV and its related conditions.

Related to:

Complex therapeutic regimens; confusing health care system; costs of therapy; side effects of therapy; interactions of therapies; knowledge deficit; decisional conflicts; mistrust of therapies and/or health care providers; questionable benefits of therapy; insufficient social support

Defining Characteristics:

Confusion and frustration over therapeutic requirements

- **Subjective Findings:** Verbalizes a desire to treat problems and prevent complications, difficulty with integration of therapies into daily life, and/or inability to complete actions required in therapy

- **Objective Findings:** Decision making that does not consider therapeutic requirements; acceleration of symptoms and/or illness

Outcome Criteria:

Active participation in health care management

Interventions	Rationales
Assess problems through an in-depth discussion with the client; identify causative and contributing factors	Provides baseline for planning interventions; many factors could be contributing to this dilemma; also see Noncompliance (Nonadherence), Decisional Conflict, Altered Thought Process, Anxiety, Fear, Hopelessness, Powerlessness, Self-Esteem Disturbance, Altered Family Process, Social Isolation, Ineffective Individual Coping, Ineffective Denial, Ineffective Family Coping (below)

Interventions	Rationales
Teach client about each therapy: ascertain client and family expectations from the therapy; discuss potential benefits and side effects; provide written schedules and guidelines for medications; demonstrate equipment and require that client and/or family member provide return demonstrations for procedures; discuss follow-up/adjunct care required (i.e., regular lab monitoring); list complications that need to be reported immediately; assist with required modifications of home and lifestyle; refer to community agencies for peer and family support	Decreases knowledge deficit; provides information needed to make decisions and initiate therapy; establishes nurse as a knowledgeable and supportive resource
Promote trust: provide information, but expect client to make decisions; use active listening skills; accept client's ambivalent feelings; help client clarify stance; be honest	Promotes security; empowers client to make and follow through on decisions

Interventions	Rationales
Encourage active participation of family and significant others if desired by the client	Supports client during implementation of therapy; decreases the risk of sabotage
Remind client that any new therapy requires behavior changes that take time to accomplish; emphasize successes; accept relapses and encourage problem solving to return to desired therapy	Decreases risk of self-blame and recriminations that may lead the client to abandon therapy
Accept changes in client's desires and plans	Demonstrates acceptance of the client as primary decision maker

Evaluation:

The client:

1. Relates less anxiety about specific therapeutic interventions
2. Discusses potential means for overcoming problems inherent in adhering to therapeutic regimen
3. Develops a plan for integrating therapies into usual living patterns
4. States intent to implement plans to integrate therapies into life

Noncompliance (Nonadherence)

A state in which the HIV-infected client desires to adhere to health care requirements but is unable to do so.

*Author's Note:

This diagnosis does not apply to the individual who chooses not to comply with recommendations of health care providers. The focus at this point is on the increasingly complicated and expensive care required.

Related to:

Side effects of therapy; frequency of clinic visits, medication dosages, and follow-up requirements; prolonged therapy required for chronic condition; costs of care; lack of support (from family, peers, employer); knowledge deficit; poor self-esteem; hopelessness; fear; anxiety; distrust of "traditional" health care system; lack of personal interactions with care providers; transportation problems; child care problems; difficulty balancing health care with other aspects of life; conflicts with personal values, cultural influences, or spiritual beliefs

Defining Characteristics:

Inconsistency between expressed desires and actions

- **Subjective Findings:** States that adherence is a problem; discusses feelings that the costs outweigh the benefits; complains about side effects

- **Objective Findings:** Observations that client is not adhering to recommendations; missed appointments; confusion; progression of disease (development of complications, exacerbation of symptoms, increases in viral loads, decreases in CD4+ T cells)

Outcome Criteria:

Decreased barriers to health care

Interventions/Rationales

See Noncompliance (Nonadherence) in Secondary Prevention; also see Ineffective Management of Therapeutic Regimen (above)

Evaluation:

The client:

1. Identifies barriers to adherence
2. Verbalizes fears, anxiety, guilt, remorse, frustration
3. Develops resources and a plan to increase ability to adhere to treatment regimens

Hyperthermia

A state in which the client's body temperature is elevated above her or his normal range.

Related to:

HIV infection; secondary infection(s); dehydration; medication reactions

Defining Characteristics:

Temperature greater than client's baseline (usually above 37.8° C/101° F orally or 38.8° C/102° F rectally)

- **Subjective Findings:** Provides history of fever, recurrent night sweats, fatigue, and malaise; reports history of vomiting, diarrhea, and/or symptoms of specific infectious processes such as coughing, headaches, sore throat, etc.

- **Objective Findings:** Elevated temperature; hot, flushed skin; diaphoresis; tachycardia; tachypnea; altered mental status including decreased levels of alertness, cognition, and orientation; dehydration manifested by dry skin, poor skin turgor, decreased fluid intake and output, concentrated urine

Outcome Criteria:

Temperature maintained within baseline norms

Interventions	Rationales
Assist in determination of cause of temperature elevation; report findings to care provider; assist in collection of laboratory specimens; refer to Introduction for treatment of HIV and opportunistic infections; refer to Fluid Volume Deficit (below) for dehydration	Identification and treatment of underlying cause of fever provides best chance for long-term solution
Provide the following interventions to decrease fever:	
Provide antipyretic medication as ordered	Acts on the hypothalamus to lower body temperature; increases comfort level through analgesic action

Interventions	Rationales
Adjust environmental factors by removing excess clothing and blankets, cooling room temperature, using fans to circulate air, changing clothes and bed clothes frequently if diaphoresis is a problem	Decreases factors that contribute to the retention of body heat; allows for convection and evaporation which contribute to the decrease in body heat; promotes comfort
Use tepid sponge baths, ice packs to groin and axilla, or hypothermia blanket to control excessively high fevers; observe for and control shivering episodes	Facilitates heat loss through convection, conduction, and evaporation; shivering increases body temperature
Maintain safety: monitor mental status and seizure activity; institute bed rest and side rails for confusion and uncoordinated motor activity; institute seizure precautions for client with history of febrile seizures or extreme temperature elevations	Neurologic function is affected by hyperthermia, infection, dehydration, and/or electrolyte imbalances, all of which may be present

Interventions	Rationales
Encourage intake of 2-3 liters of cool liquids per day	Replenishes fluid losses due to diaphoresis, hyperpnea, hyperthermia; enhances body processes that can decrease fever; prevents dehydration
Monitor vital signs every 2 hours	Assesses efficacy of interventions; allows early recognition of the development of potential complications
Teach client and/or family to monitor and treat fever at home: instruct in the use of thermometers; demonstrate record keeping; instruct in the proper use of interventions described above; define parameters for reporting to health care providers	Decreases knowledge deficit; promotes comfort and confidence in ability to maintain home care

Evaluation:

The client:

1. Maintains body temperature within normal range
2. Remains comfortable and safe during fever episode

Fluid Volume Deficit

A state in which the client experiences vascular, cellular, or intracellular dehydration.

Related to:

Nausea; vomiting; malabsorption related to HIV enteropathy; diarrhea; fever; increased metabolic rate; systemic infection(s); decreased motivation to drink fluids related to painful lesions in the mouth, depression, apathy, fatigue; anorexia; difficulty swallowing; diaphoresis

Defining Characteristics:

Negative balance of intake and output; insufficient oral intake

- **Subjective Findings:** Reports excessive vomiting, diarrhea, fever, night sweats, decreased urine output; complains of thirst, dry mouth, dry skin, dizziness or lightheadedness; complains of difficulty swallowing and/or painful lesions in mouth

- **Objective Findings:** Weight loss; signs of dehydration include the following: poor skin turgor, pallor, orthostatic hypotension, elevated temperature, tachycardia, dry skin and mucous membranes, concentrated urine, elevated specific gravity, increased hematocrit, elevated blood urea nitrogen (BUN) and creatinine values, electrolyte imbalances; untreated dehydration can lead to renal failure and circulatory collapse

Outcome Criteria:

Adequate hydration

Interventions	Rationales
Assess for signs of dehydration: weight loss, orthostatic hypotension, tachycardia, dry mucous membranes, poor skin turgor	Establishes baseline; provides opportunity for early recognition and intervention

Interventions	Rationales
Monitor intake and output	Assesses fluid balance; warns of impending problems
Monitor serum electrolytes, BUN, urine osmolality, creatinine, hematocrit, and hemoglobin; monitor blood glucose if on pentamidine	Provides baseline; detects emerging as well as existing problems; be aware that a dehydrated client with anemia may have a normal or borderline hematocrit
Encourage fluid intake of at least 2-3 liters per day; assure ready access to preferred fluids; set intake schedule; increase intake to compensate for excessive losses through vomiting, diarrhea, diaphoresis; encourage use of juices and electrolyte-rich fluids	Encourages client to participate in care; supports fluid replacement
Treat underlying problems as possible by initiating nursing and/or medical interventions for diarrhea, nausea, fever, infection, etc.	Increases ability to maintain oral intake; assists in a return to optimal fluid balance

Interventions	Rationales
Administer IV fluids and electrolytes as ordered: maintain patent IV access, monitor flow rates (rapid replacement may be required), monitor client response	Provides replacement of fluids and electrolytes
Monitor mental status, behavioral changes, level of consciousness; institute safety measures as required	Confusion and dementia symptoms can accompany dehydration; protects from injury
Provide routine skin and mouth care	Prevents breakdown; promotes comfort; allows regular assessments of skin and mucous membrane surfaces

Evaluation:

The client:

1. Replaces fluid losses
2. Maintains fluid and electrolyte balance
3. Takes in enough fluids to maintain body function
4. Demonstrates no signs or symptoms of dehydration or electrolyte imbalance

Risk for Infection

A state in which the client is at increased risk of being infected by an opportunistic or pathogenic organism.

*Author's Note:

Clients with HIV infection and AIDS are at risk for infection from both endogenous and exogenous sources, but many of the major opportunistic infections are caused by organisms that already exist in the client's body. Additional infections compound the hypermetabolism caused by HIV and, therefore, increase the strain on nutritional status, immune response, and overall ability to cope with stress.

Related to:

Cellular immune deficiency caused by the destruction of CD4+ T lymphocytes; chronic disease; use of immune suppressive substances such as tobacco, alcohol, street drugs; bone marrow suppression related to drug therapy; impaired skin and mucous membranes; periodontal disease; use of antibiotic, antiviral, antifungal, antineoplastic agents; radiation therapy; presence of invasive lines; malnutrition; stress; inadequate personal hygiene; immobility

Defining Characteristics:

Immune suppression

- **Subjective Findings:** Complains of persistent fever, night sweats, malaise, weakness, anorexia, weight loss, fatigue, headache, diarrhea, difficulty swallowing, vision changes, stiff neck, swollen lymph glands, skin or mucous membrane lesions, shortness of breath, cough, burning, itching, pain

- **Objective Findings:** Elevated temperature; weight loss; lesions of the retina, mouth, throat, vagina, rectum, penis, skin; lymphadenopathy; abdominal pain or tenderness; stiff neck; areas of congestion or consolidation over lung fields; positive cultures from various sources; CD4+

T lymphocyte counts below 500/mm³; reversed CD4:CD8 ratio

Outcome Criteria:

Remains free from opportunistic infection

Interventions	Rationales
Monitor vital signs every 2-4 hours as indicated: instruct client and family members how to monitor and document vital signs at home	Provides baseline; allows early detection of changes that may indicate a new infection; remember that sepsis may develop without fever in immune suppressed clients
Inform patient and family of signs and symptoms of infection that need to be reported to the health care provider (see Assessment, above)	Early recognition and intervention can result in easier management of infectious processes
Assist with the collection of appropriate laboratory specimens and monitor reports	Watch for positive cultures and neutropenia
Encourage immune enhancing activities related to nutrition, exercise, stress reduction, relaxation, and alterations in substance use; see Health Seeking Behaviors (above) and in Secondary Prevention	Decreases susceptibility to opportunistic disease

Interventions	Rationales
Use BSI (see Introduction) or UPs; protect client from health care workers who are potentially infectious (i.e., with weeping lesions, cold or flu symptoms, etc.)	Protects the client as well as the health care worker
Use strict aseptic technique for all invasive procedures	Prevents high-risk exposure to external organisms
Administer antimicrobials as ordered, and instruct client and family on proper techniques for at-home administration; note: a number of antimicrobials are used in HIV infection to prevent initial infection with an organism or to suppress an organism after an acute occurrence of infection (see Introduction)	Maintains adequate blood levels of the drug; decreases the risk of drug resistance; prophylactic or maintenance administration can prevent potentially life threatening episodes of acute infection
Initiate measures to prevent or compensate for dehydration (see Hypovolemia, above)	Replenishes fluid losses caused by hypermetabolism, diarrhea, vomiting, insensible loss; promotes comfort; prevents problems associated with hypovolemia

Evaluation:

The client:

1. Remains free of opportunistic infections
2. Lists signs and symptoms that need to be reported
3. Initiates steps to prevent infection

Risk for Infection Transmission

A state in which the HIV-infected client is at risk for transmitting HIV to others.

Related to:

Lack of knowledge; sharing of injection equipment; unprotected sexual intercourse; accidents in which others come into contact with client's blood; denial

Defining Characteristics:

Continued risk to others

- **Subjective Findings:** Reports unprotected sexual activity; discusses sharing equipment when injecting drugs

- **Objective Findings:** Diagnosis of HIV infection; fails to disclose HIV status to sex or drug using partner(s) and/or health care workers when appropriate

Outcome Criteria:

Decreased risk for HIV transmission

Interventions/Rationales

Initiate interventions described in Risk for Infection Transmission in Secondary Prevention.

Evaluation:

The client:

1. Lists methods in which HIV can be transmitted
2. Demonstrates activities that decrease the risk of transmission to others
3. States intent to use risk reduction measures to protect others

Altered Nutrition: Less than Body Requirements

A state in which the client experiences weight loss related to inadequate intake and/or increased metabolism of nutrients.

*Author's Note:

Wasting and malnutrition frequently accompany the progression of HIV disease. Malnutrition contributes to immune dysfunction and immune dysfunction contributes to wasting, creating a vicious downward spiral. Close attention to nutritional status can help to improve the HIV-infected client's quality of life, and may positively influence long-term survival and/or quality of life.

Related to:

Increased need for nutrient intake due to chronic infectious and/or neoplastic disease process(es); hypermetabolic state caused by infection(s), decreased ability to take food in due to mouth and esophageal lesions, nausea, vomiting, anorexia, apathy, depression; decreased ability to absorb nutrients in the GI tract; diarrhea; GI tract infections or cancers; decreased ability to obtain, prepare, or safely store food because of problems related to transportation, economics, fatigue, lack of social support, impaired cognition, immobility; knowledge deficit; side effects of medications

Defining Characteristics:

Loss of 10% or more of ideal body mass

- **Subjective Findings:** Complains of lack of appetite, altered taste sensations, discomfort when eating due to mouth sores and/or difficulty swallowing, nausea, vomiting, diarrhea, abdominal cramping; reports weight loss; provides 24 hour intake diary that reveals less than adequate intake; describes economic or psychosocial problems that decrease ability to purchase and prepare food

- **Objective Findings:** Weight loss; wasted appearance; mental confusion; oral exam reveals mouth lesions and/or advanced gingivitis; lesions in throat; abnormal bowel sounds; inability to feed self; skin, hair, and nail changes that indicate malnutrition; triceps skin fold, mid-arm circumference and mid-arm muscle circumference less than 60% of standard; muscle weakness and tenderness; knowledge deficit related to nutrition; lab work reveals decreased serum albumin levels and a negative nitrogen balance

Outcome Criteria:

Adequate nutritional intake

Interventions	Rationales	Interventions	Rationales
Assist with diagnosis of underlying problem(s); instruct client and family in appropriate use of prescribed therapies	Treatment of diagnosed problems eases discomfort and allows client to reinstitute usual eating practices; treatable problems related to nutritional deficit include HIV infection and most of the opportunistic diseases; treating the following conditions can decrease problems with ingestion: oral candidiasis, esophageal candidiasis, oral herpes simplex, acute gingivitis, oral KS; treating the following problems can decrease malabsorption and diarrhea: HIV, CMV, MAC, *Salmonella*, KS in the GI tract, *Cryptosporidium*, *Isospora belli*	Assess client's knowledge about optimal nutritional intake; ask client or family caregiver to keep a 7 day food diary to assess adequacy of intake; teach client to focus on a well-balanced diet that is high in protein and calories; encourage client to discuss dietary changes; identify and discourage use of "fad" or "miracle" diets that eliminate or severely limit major food groups, protein, or calorie intake; incorporate client's religious, social, and cultural dietary habits into nutritional plan	Identifies learning needs; supports healthy approach to nutrition; decreases likelihood of inappropriate nutritional changes that can further diminish nutritional reserves

Interventions	Rationales	Interventions	Rationales
Increase protein, calorie, and fat intake by encouraging the following techniques: add powdered milk to whole milk, cream sauces, and soups; increase intake of meats, peanut butter, and beans; add cheese to soups and vegetables; use cream or half-and-half instead of milk in soups, sauces, and milk shakes; eat hard-boiled eggs and cheeses for snacks; use extra sour cream, cream cheese, butter, sugar, honey, and mayonnaise; drink calorie-/ protein-rich nutritional supplements; eat several small meals or snacks during the day	Increases chances of meeting increased daily requirements for protein and calories	Encourage socialization with family and significant others during meals	Enhances psychosocial support; reduces stress if family supports but does not force intake; makes mealtimes more pleasant; gives client something to look forward to rather than to avoid
		Review food safety standards (see Health Seeking Behaviors in Secondary Prevention)	Prevents risk of food-borne infections
Schedule procedures, especially those that are painful, highly stressful, or nauseating, so that they do not interfere with mealtimes	Decreases unpleasant stimuli near meals; increases chances to enhance intake	Minimize factors related to anorexia: assess food likes and dislikes; aerate living areas well to prevent unpleasant odors; use spices and marinades to enhance taste of foods; encourage 6 or more small meals a day rather than 2-3 big ones; encourage rest before and after meals; if needed, provide antiemetic medications on a routine schedule prior to meals; encourage protein- and calorie-dense foods	Supports intake of nutrients when client does not feel like eating

Interventions	Rationales	Interventions	Rationales
Minimize oral and esophageal pain: teach client to avoid foods that are spicy, acidic, salty, rough in texture, excessively hot or cold, sticky; teach client to choose foods that are easy to swallow, soothing, cool or at room temperature; use popsicles to numb mouth and throat; provide oral analgesics prior to eating; encourage fluids to keep mouth moist; provide, or assist client in, good oral hygiene measures	Decreases pain associated with eating; increases palatability of food; prevents new oral infections; also see Altered Oral Mucous Membranes (below)	Help client obtain and prepare food: assess financial status and refer to social services for economic assistance as needed; evaluate home kitchen facilities (if any), and recommend ways to make food preparation more efficient; include family in dietary plans and encourage their active participation in meal planning and preparation; as needed, refer client to resources that provide alternative housing, home-maker assistance, food delivery services, etc.	Decreases risk of malnutrition related to lack of money and/or social supports
		Provide referrals to dietitians, social workers, case managers, etc., as needed	Identifies resources for the client

Interventions	Rationales
Maintain oral intake as possible; if oral intake is inadequate, discuss alternative means of nutritional intake including enteral and intravenous feeding options	Oral intake maintains GI tract function, is less invasive and less costly; alternative feeding tactics can provide essential nutrition when the client is unable to ingest foods orally; alternative methods may be used in conjunction with oral intake, in place of oral intake, or intermittently to support client during acute episodes when intake cannot be maintained

Evaluation:

The client:

1. Increases nutritional intake of proteins, calories, and micronutrients
2. Reduces weight loss
3. Regains previous weight losses
4. Maintains adequate nutritional intake for metabolic needs
5. Identifies resources that can assist with nutritional support

Impaired Swallowing

A state in which the client has decreased ability to voluntarily pass fluids and/or solid foods from the mouth to the stomach.

Related to:

Infectious and/or neoplastic lesions of the mouth, throat, esophagus; fatigue; depression

Defining Characteristics:

Difficulty or pain when swallowing

- **Subjective Findings:** Describes feeling of fullness and pain behind the sternum; refuses to eat because of pain; expresses fear at the possibility of aspiration or choking; reports coughing, choking, or other problems when swallowing

- **Objective Findings:** Decreased intake; grimaces when swallowing; weight loss; holds food or fluids in oral cavity; signs of inadequate nutritional intake

Outcome Criteria:

Decreased pain and improved ability to swallow

Interventions	Rationales
Initiate interventions described in Fluid Volume Deficit and Altered Nutrition: Less than Body Requirements (above) that are pertinent to swallowing; assist with diagnosis of underlying problem and minimize oral and esophageal pain through treatment of underlying problem and administration of analgesic medications	Identifies treatable problems; decreases discomfort of swallowing

Interventions	Rationales
Reduce possibility of aspiration: position correctly with head up; encourage use of a back-and-forth tilting motion of the head during swallowing; assure adequate time between bites	Reduces fear of aspiration
Consult speech therapy for assessment and treatment	Assures expert assistance with swallowing problems

Evaluation:

The client:

1. Reports improved ability to swallow
2. Maintains oral nutritional intake sufficient to meet metabolic needs

Impaired Skin Integrity

A state in which the client's skin is at risk of being adversely affected.

Related to:

Malnutrition, emaciation, micronutrient deficiency, dehydration, immobility and development of pressure areas, frequent diarrhea, reactions to drug or radiation therapy, dry skin, pruritus, anemia, immune deficiency, stress, poor hygiene habits; skin conditions commonly seen in HIV infection include herpes simplex, herpes zoster (shingles), psoriasis, seborrhea, candidiasis, folliculitis, bacillary angiomatosis, molluscum contagiosum, KS lesions

Defining Characteristics:

Disruptions of epidermal and dermal tissues

- **Subjective Findings:** Reports bruises, blisters, rashes, open sores, or redness on any skin surface; complains of rectal pain or discomfort; describes weight loss, diarrhea, itching, burning, edema of extremities

- **Objective Findings:** Erythematous rash, herpetic vesicles, perianal excoriation, reddened pressure points, edematous extremities, variety of lesions related to KS and/or infectious processes

Outcome Criteria:

Skin remains intact

Interventions	Rationales
Monitor status of skin on a regular basis; teach client and family to monitor skin condition at home	Provides baseline information and ability to recognize developing problems early
Teach methods to keep skin clean and well moisturized: daily shower with mild, nondrying soap; pat dry and apply emollient cream while skin is still moist; clean rectal area with warm soapy water and rinse well after each bowel movement, pat dry and apply moisturizing cream	Assists in maintenance of skin integrity

Interventions	Rationales
Alleviate itching with cool, moist compresses, topical anesthetic creams, emollient creams and lotions; discourage scratching that may extend or introduce infectious processes; administer antipruritic agents as ordered	Promotes comfort; decreases extension of problem; reduces risk of damage from scratching
Encourage ambulation or repositioning every two hours; use egg crate or sheepskin devices to protect skin while in bed	Prevents development of pressure sores
Maintain adequate hydration and nutrition (see above)	Maintains skin elasticity and function; assists to repair damage
Use aseptic technique to provide care to open wounds	Prevents introduction of pathogenic organisms

Evaluation:

The client:

1. Maintains skin integrity
2. Demonstrates ability to provide skin care
3. Experiences reduced or relieved symptoms of inflammation
4. Verbalizes increased comfort

Altered Oral Mucous Membranes

A state in which the client experiences change or disruption to the oral mucous membranes.

*Author's Note:

Oral care should receive high priority for all HIV-infected clients. Maintaining oral health helps to prevent pain, insults to body image, oral infections, gingivitis, and the need for difficult interventions. Oral health is also a primary factor in maintaining adequate nutrition and hydration.

Related to:

Opportunistic diseases including candidiasis, herpes simplex, oral hairy leukoplakia, KS; primary HIV infection; poor oral hygiene; overgrowth of normal flora; malnutrition; dehydration; reactions to drug or local radiation therapy; periodontal disease; continued use of alcohol and tobacco; mouth breathing related to nasal and sinus infections; knowledge and/or skill deficits to perform appropriate mouth care

Defining Characteristics:

Disrupted oral mucous membranes

- **Subjective Findings:** Complains of dryness, bleeding, soreness, or burning in mouth or throat; reports changes in taste, pain when eating, or difficulty swallowing; reveals variety of lesions or inflamed areas in oral cavity; verbalizes difficulty in eating spicy or salty foods

- **Objective Findings:** Variety of lesions in oral cavity such as white patchy areas, red-purple raised lesions, bleeding and inflamed gums, loose or missing teeth; halitosis; dry, cracked lips; diagnostic tests can provide identification of source of a number of pathogens or KS; enlarged lymph nodes in the neck

Outcome Criteria:

Intact oral mucous membranes that are free from irritation and pain

Interventions	Rationales
Initiate prophylactic measures to prevent or decrease the emergence of oral problems; see Health Seeking Behavior in Secondary Prevention	Reduces risk of oral problems thus saving the client pain, inconvenience, and expense; assists in maintaining adequate nutritional intake
Monitor condition of oral cavity on a routine basis	Identifies problems early and allows initiation of treatment; provides basis for education about oral hygiene

Interventions	Rationales
Teach client and/or family how to perform good oral hygiene; provide oral hygiene if client or family is unable to do so; include the following methods: use a soft toothbrush and nonabrasive toothpaste; if mouthwash is desired, select one without alcohol; brush teeth at least twice a day and preferably after every meal; floss teeth at least once a day; provide meticulous care for dentures or other oral appliances	Prevents gum and mouth diseases; promotes comfort; improves halitosis; removes debris that can support organism growth; removes plaque that causes gingivitis; freshens mouth; stimulates appetite
Encourage frequent rinsing of mouth with saline solution or Peridex	Maintains oral hygiene between brushing; decreases dryness; Peridex has qualities that help prevent gingivitis
Apply moisturizer to lips as often as needed	Promotes comfort; decreases dryness and painful cracking of lips
Administer topical antibiotics and/or analgesia as ordered; teach client to avoid oral intake for 30 minutes after application	Treats underlying cause; promotes healing and comfort

Interventions	Rationales
Assist client to alter diet for comfort by avoiding spicy and salty foods; avoiding extremely hot or cold foods; encouraging foods with soft, creamy textures	Prevents irritation; encourages maintenance of adequate nutritional intake
Encourage fluid intake of 2-3 liters per day; keep preferred fluids readily available; provide hourly reminders to drink; keep an intake chart to monitor oral fluids	Prevents dehydration; promotes comfort in oral cavity
Discourage continued use of tobacco and alcohol	Decreases drying, oral lesions, oral pathology, and infection related to use of these agents
Encourage routine dental care every 3 months by a dentist who is knowledgeable in caring for HIV-infected clients	Prevents oral problems; allows for early recognition and treatment of emerging problems; provides therapy needed after problems occur

Evaluation:

The client:

1. Demonstrates ability to perform appropriate oral care
2. Describes oral pathology that needs to be reported to health care providers
3. Experiences maximum oral comfort
4. Maintains intact mucous membranes
5. Receives care to treat oral problems

Altered Bowel Elimination: Diarrhea

A state in which the client experiences a change in normal bowel habits, characterized by the frequent passage of loose, fluid, unformed stools.

Related to:

Gastrointestinal infections caused by HIV, *Giardia lamblia, Salmonella, Shigella, Campylobacter, Isospora belli, Cryptosporidium, Mycobacterium avium* complex, CMV, herpes simplex, or any other common GI tract pathogen; KS lesions in the GI tract; lactose intolerance; nutritional problems; intolerance to dietary supplements with a high osmolarity (either by mouth or NG tube); gastritis; irritable bowel; side effect to drug or radiation therapy

Defining Characteristics:

Frequent expulsion of loose or liquid stool

- **Subjective Findings:** Complains of passing loose stools frequently during the day, abdominal pain, cramping, or urgency; reports weakness, lack of appetite, and signs of dehydration; discusses problems with incontinence and fears of being too far from a bathroom for easy access; reports changes in social activities because of fear of diarrhea

- **Objective Findings:** Signs of dehydration; electrolyte imbalances; tenderness on abdominal palpation; hyperactive bowel sounds; documentation of stool losses of up to 12 liters of fluid per day; perianal excoriation; stool examination may provide diagnosis of pathogens

Outcome Criteria:

Control of diarrhea and the complications of diarrhea

Interventions	Rationales	Interventions	Rationales
Assess elimination patterns and document quality, quantity, frequency of stools; observe for blood, fat, or undigested food in stool	Provides baseline; assists in differential diagnosis; facilitates selection of appropriate therapy	Assess perianal area and initiate skin care measures to prevent/treat problems by cleaning rectal area thoroughly with Tucks or baby wipes after each stool, and applying creams or ointments that soothe and provide continued protection	Prevents skin breakdown, pain, and pruritus; assists in odor control
Assess and monitor bowel sounds	Hyperactive bowel sounds are common		
Monitor intake and output, vital signs, daily weight, evidence of hypovolemia	Provides early recognition and intervention for hypovolemia, which, if left untreated, can cause inadequate tissue perfusion, renal dysfunction, and/or circulatory collapse	Teach clients to use incontinence pads or pants to protect clothing in case of incontinence	Decreases risk of embarrassing incidences; encourages client to continue social activities
		Monitor stool culture and/or intestinal biopsy results	Identifies causative factors and assists with initiation of appropriate therapy
Initiate intervention to prevent dehydration and malnutrition discussed in Fluid Volume Deficit and Altered Nutrition: Less than Body Requirements (above); encourage daily intake of 2-3 liters of fluids (especially juices and electrolyte-rich products); introduce lactose-free diet if lactose intolerance is diagnosed; encourage low-residue, high-protein, high-calorie diet; involve dietitian and family in discussions of dietary changes	Decreases risk of harmful consequences of prolonged diarrhea	Administer anti-diarrheal agents on a routine schedule rather than PRN, especially during times of acute diarrheal episodes	Controls diarrhea more consistently; assists in prevention of fluid losses
		Encourage client to discuss psychosocial problems related to diarrhea	Allows assessment and development of interventions that may assist client to continue usual activities; allows discussion of embarrassing problem; supports client and promotes holistic care

Evaluation:

The client:

1. Experiences reduced frequency of stools
2. Maintains intact skin and mucous membranes in perianal region
3. Maintains adequate hydration, nutrition, and comfort levels
4. Maintains usual social activities

Activity Intolerance

A state in which the client has insufficient energy to complete required or desired daily activities.

Related to:

Weakness; fatigue; CNS and peripheral neurologic involvement; respiratory problems; malnutrition; fluid and electrolyte imbalances; anemia; diarrhea; prolonged immobility; chronic disease; infectious and neoplastic processes; side effects to medications; depression; sense of futility; stress; pain; sleep disturbances

Defining Characteristics:

Altered physiologic response to activity

- **Subjective Findings:** Complains of weakness, fatigue, shortness of breath, malaise; verbalizes frustration over inability to complete normal and/or desired activities; reports problems with ambulation, coordination, and balance; refuses to participate in usual activities; feels exhausted after activity

- **Objective Findings:** Appearance of fatigue and energy depletion; moves slowly and may be uncoordinated; requires considerable assistance for routine activities such as ambulation, eating, bathing, and dressing, muscle atrophy; wasting

Outcome Criteria:

Endurance and energy levels sufficient to perform activities of daily living (ADLs)

Interventions	Rationales
Minimize contributing factors, see the following: Hyperthermia, Fluid Volume Deficit, Risk for Infection, Altered Nutrition: Less than Body Requirements, Altered Bowel Elimination: Diarrhea (above), and Altered Respiratory Function, Sleep Pattern Disturbance, Pain, Anxiety, Fatigue, Fear, Hopelessness, Powerlessness, Grieving, Social Isolation, Altered Sexuality Patterns, Ineffective Individual Coping, and Spiritual Distress (below)	Deals with underlying problems that contribute to activity intolerance; allows energy restoration and comfort

Interventions	Rationales
Initiate plans to conserve and enhance energy: efficient positioning of most-needed items, furniture, etc.; encourage rest before and after periods of activity; use shower chair during bathing and routine hygiene activities; make use of frozen foods and microwave ovens as possible; develop routine schedule that allows for periods of uninterrupted rest	Conserves energy; acknowledges difficulties in performing actions
Discuss need to start considering changes in work activities, decreasing hours for example	Assists client to begin considering long-term implications of HIV disease, activity intolerance, and fatigue
Provide care that the client cannot do for self; teach family members to provide supportive care as needed; if energy losses are temporary, return responsibilities to client gradually as energy levels increase	Reassures client that care will be provided as his or her abilities decrease; promotes comfort

Interventions	Rationales
Refer, as needed, to physical therapy, occupational therapy, or exercise physiology	Provides specialized input and care planning consultation
Encourage family and significant others to participate in care plans and interventions for activity intolerance; encourage them to provide assistance when needed and to support planned interventions	Assures client of needed assistance; encourages client to adhere to intervention plans that increase tolerance, schedule rest and activities, and support nutritional and exercise programs

Evaluation:

The client:

1. Develops increased tolerance for activity
2. Utilizes scheduling and assistive devices to compensate for lack of energy
3. Verbalizes a decrease in frustration related to activity intolerance

Impaired Home Maintenance Management

A state in which the individual and/or family is unable to independently maintain a safe, care-providing environment for the HIV-infected client.

*Author's Note:

Home health care is an ideal setting for health maintenance for HIV-infected clients who frequently do not need intensive, acute, or chronic institutionalized care. In ideal situations, home care promotes independence, self-esteem, and family involvement. It must be noted, however, that many HIV-infected clients do not have ideal living situations. Some are homeless, some have less than adequate housing or support, and some are simply unable to continue in their present situations. Clients with child care responsibilities will need assistance for their children as well. (See Parental Role Conflict below.) Nursing assessment, intervention, referral, and creativity are essential to help clients receive optimal healthcare in an appropriate setting.

Related to:

Activity intolerance; chronic, debilitating disease; financial problems; lack of information about local resources; self-care deficit; inadequate support system; impaired mental status; substance use; inadequate housing or furnishings; inadequate community services

Defining Characteristics:

Inadequate home environment for appropriate health maintenance

- **Subjective Findings:** Verbalizes difficulty in maintaining housekeeping, a safe environment, home repair; discusses financial difficulties related to housing; reports lack of assistance at home; complains of fatigue or weakness; demonstrates inadequate knowledge or skills to administer medications and prescribed treatments

- **Objective Findings:** Observations that indicate problems with maintaining a safe, clean environment; demonstrated inability to care for self in home and/or to complete activities of daily living; lack of connection with local resources and support systems; lack of adequate safety devices such as ramps and handrails; lack of adequate heating, cooling, lighting, kitchen, or bathroom facilities; absence of transportation; dirty environment and/or the presence of insects or rodents; dangerous neighborhood

Outcome Criteria:

Improved home environment which promotes health maintenance

Interventions	Rationales
Assess abilities to maintain health in the current home environment: status of housing related to cleanliness, safety, adequate kitchen and bathroom facilities, etc.; client's ability to provide for self-care in current housing, willingness, and availability of family/significant others to provide needed supports; reassess on a regular basis because client's health status, the ability to care for self, the ability to maintain housing, and the availability of supportive others can change over time; listen to realities of the home situation	Provides baseline; allows early recognition of problematic changes; findings will guide interventions

Interventions	Rationales	Interventions	Rationales
Discuss changes in functional capacity that will require lifestyle changes with the client and, if acceptable to the client, with family/significant others: identify care needs related to nutrition, hygiene, nursing, or other professional services, finances, transportation, childcare, etc.	Initiates discussion of perceived needs for assistance; identifies areas of concern that will direct future discussions	Determine need for durable medical equipment and supplies (oxygen, IV equipment, bedside commodes, walkers, hospital beds, etc.); order equipment and arrange for delivery; teach client or family members proper and safe use of the equipment; ask for return demonstration of equipment use	Ensures adequate equipment to maintain care at home; promotes safe and effective use of equipment
Make appropriate referrals to case management, social services, and/or home health agencies for homemakers and nursing services, transportation and nutritional assistance programs, HIV/AIDS community-based organizations, childcare support systems; if needed, refer to community-based housing for HIV-infected clients (if available) or alternative housing arrangements	Initiates services through community agencies; provides financial, medical, nursing, social, nutritional, and transportation needs to allow continued independence at home	Encourage family/significant other participation: teach basics of care and nutrition; teach and encourage use of BSI; review appropriate responses to emergency situations; provide respite care and referrals for emotional support; encourage family members to support maximal independence for the client for as long as possible	The availability of willing and knowledgeable family members often makes the difference in the ability to maintain home care; provides family with knowledge and support to continue care; acknowledges their importance to the client and home care; decreases family anxiety; promotes independence and client-focused care

Evaluation:

The client or family/significant other:

1. Demonstrates ability to access supports needed to continue health care maintenance in the home
2. Demonstrates skills required to continue care in the home
3. Requests and receives necessary assistance
4. Expresses satisfaction with housing, support services, and home situation
5. Maintains adequate care for dependent children

Risk for Altered Respiratory Function

A state in which the client is at risk of experiencing an imbalance in oxygen uptake and carbon dioxide elimination related to problems with the passage of air through the respiratory tract and/or to the exchange of gases at the alveolar level.

Related to:

Opportunistic infections, including PCP, CMV, *Cryptococcus neoformans*, MAC, *Mycobacterium tuberculosis, Histoplasma capsulatum, Candida albicans, Cryptosporidium*; opportunistic cancers such as KS and lymphoma; anemia; increased secretions; hypoxemia; cough; immobility; lung field radiation; anxiety; post-bronchoscopy symptoms; pain; excessive or thick secretions; analgesics; narcotics; sedatives; smoking; exercise intolerance

Defining Characteristics:

Inadequate oxygenation

- **Subjective Findings:** Complains of shortness of breath, especially related to usual levels of exercise and/or completion of ADLs; describes persistent or uncomfortable cough, fever, and/or fatigue

- **Objective Findings:** Dyspnea; rapid, shallow respirations; increased breathing effort; elevated temperature; decreased, distant, or nonuniformity of breath sounds over lung fields; use of accessory muscles for respiration; circumoral cyanosis; CXR shows infiltrates or miliary pattern; sputum cultures reveal pathogenic organisms; lung biopsy reveals pathogenic organism or malignancy; arterial blood gases (ABGs) reveal hypoxia, hypercapnia, and acid-base imbalances; decreased hematocrit and hemoglobin levels; signs of altered mentation such as confusion, somnolence, restlessness, irritability; inability to move secretions

Outcome Criteria:

Maintenance of adequate oxygen and carbon dioxide levels and return to baseline respiratory function

Interventions	Rationales
Assess and monitor respiratory status: listen to breath sounds, observe respiratory patterns and use of accessory muscles, note anxiety or effort with breathing; assess for changes in mental status or level of consciousness; assess skin color and capillary refill	Establishes baseline; detects respiratory complications

Interventions	Rationales	Interventions	Rationales
Teach client and/or family members to report problems with respiration including cough, progressive dyspnea, activity intolerance, fever	Encourages early reporting; increases chance of early intervention	Administer humidified oxygen as ordered and monitor effectiveness	Reduces risk of hypoxemia
Provide adequate hydration (2-3 liters of fluid a day); see Fluid Volume Deficit (above)	Keeps secretions liquified for easier removal	Administer anti-infectives, expectorants, and antitussives as ordered and monitor response	Facilitates resolution of pulmonary infection; promotes secretion removal
Encourage pulmonary hygiene: ambulate frequently and/or change bed position every 2 hours; teach pursed lip breathing; develop routine regimen of deep breathing and coughing; teach client to splint chest to decrease coughing pain; provide chest physiotherapy, postural drainage, and suctioning as needed	Mobilizes secretions; aids in opening airways; improves lung expansion	Assess risk of exposure to TB in the past; assess for history of TB that may become reactivated by performing TB skin testing or CXR as indicated and monitoring results	Increases chance of early discovery of active TB infection; enhances effect of intervention
		Teach energy-conserving activities; see Activity Intolerance (above) and Fatigue (below)	Assists in energy conservation; decreases oxygen use
Position to enhance ventilatory capacity: lie with good lung down, prone, or semi-Fowler's positions	Enhances lung expansion and ease of breathing	Teach relaxation techniques; see Anxiety (below)	Minimizes risk of hyperventilation related to anxiety, which will increase respiratory effort and problems with acid-base balance

Interventions	Rationales
Encourage cessation or moderation of smoking behaviors: refer to smoking cessation program; encourage daily reduction in the number of cigarettes smoked; encourage use of filtered products; discourage smoking before eating, and before, during, and immediately after performing ADLs	Decreases deleterious effects of smoking, including risk of infections and malignancies, cough, appetite suppression, activity intolerance, difficult respirations

Evaluation:

The client:

1. Describes respiratory conditions that need to be reported to the health care provider
2. Maintains optimal respiratory status
3. Verbalizes increased comfort with respiratory function and decreased problems with cough

Instrumental Self-Care Deficit

A state in which the client experiences a decreased ability to perform activities or access services needed to maintain a household.

Related to:

Muscular weakness; lack of coordination; neuromuscular disorders; visual disorders related to CMV, herpes simplex, or other organisms; depression; fatigue; immobility; neurocognitive deficits; use of medical devices including equipment for intravenous fluids and medications, feeding tubes, long-term venous access devices; inadequate support systems

Defining Characteristics:

Inability to maintain independence in home setting without assistance

- **Subjective Findings:** Verbalizes fears about maintaining self at home, especially related to food preparation, shopping, house cleaning, laundry, money management, safety, childcare, transportation, and medication administration

- **Objective Findings:** Weakness; confusion; lack of social and economic supports; lack of hygienic living conditions; lack of appropriate kitchen or bathroom facilities; nonadherence to medication regimen; missed clinic appointments; failure to safely care for children

Outcome Criteria:

Safe and effective management of at-home care

Interventions	Rationales
Assess for causative and contributing factors such as visual deficits, impaired cognition, impaired mobility, fatigue, lack of knowledge, lack of financial capabilities, lack of social support systems, inadequate housing	Provides focus for interventions

Interventions	Rationales	Interventions	Rationales
Teach methods of medication administration; provide written materials for future reference; encourage use of memory devices such as 7-day pill holders	Provides knowledge base for maintenance of therapeutic drug intake; see Noncompliance (Nonadherence) in Secondary Prevention	Encourage involvement of family members and significant others in home care; also see Ineffective Management of Therapeutic Regimen, Noncompliance (Nonadherence), Impaired Home Maintenance Management (above)	Promotes ability to maintain household
Teach methods needed to maintain equipment and access lines for IV administration	Involves client in self-care; increases self-confidence; assures proper care		
Refer to financial and social services, home health, case management, childcare assistance, and legal supports	Assures adequate funding for necessary nutritional and medical maintenance; assists with provisions of nursing care and/or homemaker services in the home; allows frequent assessment of home environment that may lead to increased at-home services; supports independent living situation; enhances appropriate planning for childcare		

Evaluation:

The client:

1. Adheres to medication regimen
2. Reports adequate nutritional intake
3. Verbalizes feelings of safety and comfort in home setting
4. Demonstrates ability to manage home environment and financial matters independently or with the assistance of others
5. Appropriately assesses need for assistance and contacts resources

Sleep Pattern Disturbance

A state in which disturbances in the quantity or quality of rest patterns causes discomfort or interferes with the client's desired lifestyle.

Related to:

Anxiety; pain; diarrhea; night sweats; chills; treatment schedules; respiratory or circulatory disorders; bladder infections with associated frequency or incontinence; immobility; medications (especially sedatives, hypnotics, antidepressants, tranquilizers, amphetamines, corticosteroids, decongestants, caffeine, alcohol); lack of exercise or change in activity pattern; lifestyle disruptions (related to occupational, social, sexual, financial, or emotional issues); environmental changes such as living conditions, living companions, moving to a new environment, etc.; stress; depression; changes in sleeping routines

Defining Characteristics:

Difficulty falling or remaining asleep

- **Subjective Findings:** Complains of difficulty in falling asleep, staying asleep, fatigue on awakening, not feeling rested, general fatigue; discusses problems with energy levels and staying awake during the day

- **Objective Findings:** Agitation, mood alterations; increasing irritability; decreased attention span; disorientation; lethargy; listlessness; decreased social interaction; frequent yawning; drooping eyelids and posture

Outcome Criteria:

Adequate rest

Interventions	Rationales
Assess problem by asking open-ended questions such as, "Describe problems you have with sleep"; "Describe the last good night's sleep that you had"; "What helps you get to sleep?"; "What causes you the most problems after you have been asleep for a while?"; determine client's usual sleep pattern before development of the current problem	Establishes baseline for intervention
Provide specific interventions for identified problems (i.e., anxiety, night sweats, use of caffeine, interruptions for medications or treatments, diarrhea, etc.)	Provides basis for targeted interventions; refer to specific nursing diagnoses to develop care plan: also see Hyperthermia, Altered Bowel Elimination: Diarrhea (above), and Pain, Anxiety, Grieving, Spiritual Distress (below)
Remind the client that there is an increased need for rest during periods of acute illness and that naps may be required during the day to reach optimal sleep requirements	Increases knowledge level; provides permission to sleep during the day for clients who do not want to appear "lazy"

Interventions	Rationales
Provide periods of stimulating activity during the day	Enhances tiredness and need for rest
Discuss sleep promoting measures: encourage usual bedtime routines; assess need for muscle relaxation techniques, back rubs, positioning, affective touch, presence; encourage the development of an established pre-sleep routine	Promotes sleep; reduces anxiety; encourages self-efficacy
Provide and maintain a calm, quiet, darkened environment	Enhances chances of uninterrupted rest
Plan rest periods of at least 90 minutes for all sleep including naps and night time sleep: arrange medications and treatments to prevent interruption of this cycle; accomplish as many needed interventions (i.e., vital signs, medications, treatments) as possible during each wake period; use flashlight for night time checks	Promotes REM sleep; assists in equilibrating normal sleep time

Interventions	Rationales
Administer sleeping or antianxiety medications as ordered; monitor effects of medication on sleep and client's perceptions of feeling rested	Some of these medications increase sleeping problems; allows for early recognition of problems and trials of alternative medications until an optimal product is prescribed

Evaluation:

The client:

1. Describes activities that can enhance sleep and rest
2. Obtains adequate rest to balance energy needs
3. Expresses satisfaction with sleep patterns

Pain

A state in which the client experiences and reports the presence of severe discomfort and/or uncomfortable sensations.

*Author's Note:

Pain is a common problem associated with HIV infection and AIDS, especially during acute episodes of opportunistic diseases. Clients with a history of drug use present a particularly difficult problem. Some of these clients are in recovery through Twelve Step Programs that discourage the use of any potentially addicting substance. These clients may refuse pharmacologic interventions because of the fear of returning to an addicted state. Other clients are willing to use medications for pain relief, but their health care providers are hesitant to use narcotics because of the known history. Frequently, clients who have used drugs in the past are under-medicated in an attempt to prevent substance abuse. The problem is that these clients, because of increased tolerance levels, will actually need more of a given drug to achieve pain relief. These are difficult issues that are best treated in a multidisciplinary team with input from specialists in addiction medicine.

Related to:

Opportunistic infections and malignancies; lymphadenopathy; edema and pressure; side effects of therapies, especially radiation and drug-related peripheral neuropathy; arthralgia; myalgia; vasculitis; inflammation; chronic demyelinating neuropathy

Defining Characteristics:

Subjective experience of pain

- **Subjective Findings:** Verbal expressions of pain: pain is what, where, and how often the client says it is; complains of headaches, muscle aches, stiff neck, cramping abdominal pain, irritation around mucous membrane lesions

- **Objective Findings:** Protective or guarding behaviors such as splinting and posture; self-focused; altered perceptions of time and space; social withdrawal; impaired thought processes; moaning, crying, whimpering, pacing, restlessness, irritability; facial features including grimacing, clenched teeth, clenched jaw, knotted brow; muscle tension; changes in blood pressure, pulse, respirations; diaphoresis; dilated pupils

Outcome Criteria:

Pain relieved, controlled, or eliminated

Interventions	Rationales
Perform comprehensive assessment of pain, preferably at a time when pain is not severe: location, character, onset, duration, frequency, quality, intensity or severity (ask to rate intensity on a scale of 1 - 10), effectiveness of pain control measures used in the past, family and cultural expectations about pain, previous experiences with pain, personal meanings of pain; observe for nonverbal cues to pain (caution: these cues are frequently influenced by the client's culture and family, the nurse must learn how each individual client expresses pain)	Identifies client perceptions of pain; assists client to verbalize experiences and meaning of pain; initiates differential diagnostic process; provides opportunity for self-assessment and the development of coping mechanism
Assist the client to identify precipitating factors to pain (i.e., fear, anxiety, lack of information, stress, specific types of activity, specific medications or treatments, etc.); develop interventions that circumvent, moderate, or eliminate these factors	Focuses on specific problems that are thought to cause problems; see Hyperthermia, Impaired Skin Integrity, Altered Oral Mucous Membranes, Altered Bowl Elimination: Diarrhea, Altered Respiratory Function (above), and Anxiety, Fatigue, Fear, Hopelessness, Powerlessness, Grieving (below)

Interventions	Rationales
Relate acceptance of client's pain through the following therapeutic communication strategies: acknowledge the presence of pain, listen attentively to discussions about the pain, convey a concern based on a desire to understand the pain, establish commitment to continue efforts to decrease pain until comfort is achieved	Decreases feelings of shame, anger or defensiveness related to pain (many clients, especially those with a history of substance use, have experienced skepticism from health care providers), assures client that s/he will not be abandoned if initial attempts to control pain are not successful; encourages client to not give up on pain relief efforts
Provide optimal pain relief with prescribed medications and monitor efficacy; encourage use of analgesics on a routine, rather than PRN basis to control pain; provide analgesia 20-30 minutes prior to painful procedures; encourage client to request pain medications before pain becomes severe; evaluate effect of medication on pain 30 minutes after administration of medication; allow client control of dosing schedules as much as possible	Promotes optimal use of analgesic medications; provides early assessment of efficacy; alerts health care providers of need to alter medication, dose, and/or schedule of administration, promotes self-care for pain control

Interventions	Rationales
Teach and encourage the use of the following nonpharmacologic methods of pain moderation (which can be used alone or in conjunction with medications): relaxation, guided imagery, warm baths, massage, moist heat or cold packs as indicated, distraction, meditation, music therapy, art therapy, humor, accupressure, therapeutic touch, biofeedback, hypnosis, spirituality, etc.; assess effect on pain	Enhances efforts to control pain; alters perceptions of pain; maintains client self-efficacy; provides alternative or supplemental support to medications
Promote adequate sleep and rest during pain-free intervals	Increases ability to cope with pain; see Sleep Pattern Disturbance (above)

Evaluation:

The client:

1. Identifies precipitating or aggravating factors to pain and develops coping mechanisms to moderate these experiences
2. Uses preferred nonpharmacologic mechanisms to assist with pain relief
3. Discusses episodes of pain with the nurse
4. Uses prescribed pain medications effectively
5. Verbalizes a decrease in the intensity and duration of pain episodes

Decisional Conflict

A state of indecision between competing choices that involve risk, loss, or challenge to established personal lifestyle or values.

Related to:

Confusing, inconsistent, or incomplete information related to HIV infection, opportunistic diseases, treatment options, legal and social issues; disagreement within support system about best course(s) to take; risks related to the potential loss of relationships, employment, health, personal control; inexperience in decision making; unclear personal value system or a conflict with personal values; ethical dilemmas related to sexuality or drug use; resignation; hopelessness

Defining Characteristics:

Vacillation between choices; delayed decision making

- **Subjective Findings:** Verbalizes uncertainty and negative consequences of perceived alternatives; expresses distress related to advancing health problems and disabilities; discusses frustrations related to health care providers' demands for decisions; examines personal values and beliefs related to quality and quantity of life; repeatedly asks for input and opinions

- **Objective Findings:** Physical signs of stress and tension; behaviors that are counter to expressed goals; unrealistic expectations; confusion; lack of information or previous experience with treatment regimens; experimental nature of many treatment options; delays in decision making; vacillation between potential choices; seeks second and third opinions

Outcome Criteria:

Effective, informed decisions

Interventions/Rationales

Initiate interventions described in Decisional Conflict in Secondary Prevention

Evaluation:

The client:

1. States advantages and disadvantages of potential choices
2. Discusses fears and concerns about choices
3. Makes and implements informed choices
4. Expresses satisfaction with decision(s)

Sensory-Perceptual Alteration

A state in which the individual experiences a change in the amount or patterning of incoming stimuli accompanied by a diminished, exaggerated, distorted, or impaired response to stimuli.

*Author's Note:

In clients with HIV infection, the most common sensory-perceptual deficits are in the areas of vision and hearing. Kinesthetic, tactile, gustatory, and olfactory problems may also occur.

Related to:

CMV retinitis; otic infections or cancers; infections and cancers of the CNS; HIV's direct effect on the peripheral nervous system; side effects to prescribed, over-the-counter, or street drugs, including hearing losses, peripheral neuropathy, disorientation, and kinesthetic problems; fluid and electrolyte imbalances caused by excessive vomiting, diarrhea, or diaphoresis; impaired oxygen transport secondary to pulmonary infections; anemia; sedatives, tranquilizers, amphetamines, hallucinogenic drugs; fatigue or other mobility restrictions; social isolation; pain, stress; sleep deprivation related to night sweats, anxiety, depression, frequent treatments, pain, etc.; fear; bereavement; change in environment (such as hospitalization for an acute episode or moving to a downstairs bedroom); dementia

Defining Characteristics:

Inability to accurately interpret environment related to problems in receiving or perceiving stimuli

- **Subjective Findings:** Complains of problems related to vision, hearing, tasting, smelling, feeling, balance, or movement; describes visual or auditory illusions or hallucinations; expresses anxiety and fear; complains of boredom, fatigue, or sleep pattern disturbances; expresses feelings of apathy or lack of concern

- **Objective Findings:** Motor incoordination; decreased abilities in the areas of seeing, hearing, moving, sensing; disorientation to time, place, or person; decreased problem-solving ability; inability to concentrate; bizarre or paranoid thinking; exaggerated emotional responses; rapid mood swings; flattened affect; anger; irritability; daydreaming; altered communication patterns; altered sleep patterns

Outcome Criteria:

Improved ability to interpret environment; no injuries related to deficits

Interventions	Rationales
Perform baseline assessment for the following: neurological function, focusing on sensory system including vision, hearing, tactile sensation, superficial pain, vibration, and proprioception; mental status including general appearance and behavior, sensorium, mood and affect, thought content, and intellectual capacity; and environment, including usual levels of stimulation, changes in levels of stimulation and social interactions; solicit input from client and significant others about changes in ability to sense and perceive the environment	Provides baseline information for the development of intervention plans

Interventions	Rationales
Determine related problems and institute appropriate interventions: see Fluid Volume Deficit, Altered Bowel Elimination: Diarrhea, Altered Respiratory Function, Sleep Pattern Disturbance, Pain (above), and Altered Thought Process, Anxiety, Fatigue, Fear, Hopelessness, Powerlessness, Grieving, Impaired Social Interaction, Social Isolation, and Spiritual Distress (below); report sensory-perceptual changes to care provider for diagnosis and treatment of infectious, neoplastic, or drug-related conditions	Initiates appropriate therapeutic interventions that can positively influence sensory and perceptual capabilities

Interventions	Rationales
Provide frequent orientation cues for the client: identify self with each interaction; address the client by name; place calendars, clocks, and familiar objects in close proximity; maintain as near to the usual environment as possible (home care, liberal visitation if hospitalization is required, use of personal toiletries and clothing, etc.); orient to new environment, personnel, treatments, etc.; avoid novelty and surprise (keep client oriented and informed of new elements in his or her care)	Assists client to compensate for losses and changes in life
Control extraneous stimuli by decreasing unfamiliar noise, traffic, and personnel; increasing use of meaningful sensations such as music, significant others, pets, familiar objects, and foods	Strives to promote meaningful stimuli while decreasing confusing input

Interventions	Rationales	Interventions	Rationales
Encourage client to discuss unusual sensations, clarify misinterpretations, discuss feelings that are caused by these sensations; refer problems as needed to other members of the health care team	Provides additional assessment; allows reorientation and opportunity to decrease anxiety and fears caused by strange sensations	*For olfactory problems:* identify and try to eliminate odors that are noxious to the client; encourage use of personal toiletries that are familiar and smell pleasant to the client; aerate room well, especially after diarrhea, vomiting, or the production of other unpleasant odors; serve foods hot when they are more apt to have a distinguishing smell; serve food that is visually appealing to compensate for decreased ability to smell; also see Altered Nutrition: Less than Body Requirements (above)	Enhances pleasant odors and ability to smell
Provide appropriate safety measures such as assistive devices, bed rails, low heeled sturdy shoes; remove throw rugs, orient to location, etc.	Decreases risk of injury		
For visual impairment: discuss treatment options and support client decisions about therapy; provide consistency in object placement and re-orient to placement as needed; enhance alternative sensory input (auditory, tactile, etc.); describe movements and intentions prior to performing any activity (especially one that requires touching the client) and on entering and leaving the room	Increases security in the environment; decreases risk of injury; decreases risk of startling the client		

Interventions	Rationales	Interventions	Rationales
For gustatory problems: provide a variety of condiments to enhance food taste; serve foods that are appealing to the client; serve foods spaced away from ingestion of unpleasant-tasting medications; serve food that is visually appealing to compensate for decreased ability to taste; alleviate dry mouth, which enhances taste sensations, by providing frequent normal saline mouth washes and avoiding mouth washes with alcohol or lemon juice; encourage client to quit or decrease use of cigarettes or alcoholic beverages; also see Altered Oral Mucous Membranes (above); use good oral hygiene measures; also see Altered Nutrition: Less than Body Requirements (above)	Compensates for changes in taste; decreases dryness of mouth	*For tactile and kinesthetic problems:* assess extent of problem and provide for safety measures that may include assistive walking devices, assistance with ambulation, low-heeled sturdy shoes, etc.; sensations such as itching, burning, or pain may be relieved with cool compresses and distraction as well as soothing lotions and analgesic or antipruritic medications; encourage frequent position changes to prevent skin breakdown; also see Impaired Skin Integrity (above); provide appropriate touch, including massage, to provide alternative tactile stimulation; encourage use of personal clothing and bed clothes that have a familiar tactile sensation for the client	Provides for safety; prevents skin breakdown; enhances comfort

Evaluation:

The client:

1. Remains safe within the environment
2. Demonstrates an improvement in orientation to person, place, and time
3. Seeks clarification regarding unusual or unpleasant sensory or perceptual events
4. Verbalizes increased comfort with ability to compensate for sensory-perceptual problems

Altered Thought Process

A state in which the client experiences a disruption in cognitive operations and activities.

Related to:

CNS infection with HIV resulting in AIDS dementia complex (ADC); aseptic meningitis; opportunistic infections of the CNS such as toxoplasmosis, CMV, HSV, VZV; progressive multifocal leukoencephalopathy (PML), cryptococcosis, histoplasmosis, mycobacterium, neurosyphilis; CNS malignancies including primary lymphoma of the brain; hypoxemia related to pulmonary impairment; drug reactions; reactions to radiation therapy; depression or anxiety; fever; stress; substance use; fear; actual or anticipated loss; emotional trauma; isolation; unclear communication; dehydration and/or nutritional deficits; electrolyte or acid-base imbalances; sensory overload or deprivation; social isolation

Defining Characteristics:

Inaccurate interpretation of internal or external stimuli

- **Subjective Findings:** Discusses altered sleep patterns; describes periods of forgetfulness, disorientation, memory loss, inability to concentrate, decreased problem-solving ability; complains of headache, stiff neck, fever, malaise; reports delusions, illusions, or hallucinations; discusses loss of interest in usual activities

- **Objective Findings:** Disoriented to person, place, time; altered levels of consciousness; impaired memory; attention deficit; hyperactivity; inappropriate or fantasy-based thinking; disturbed thought flow; disturbed thought content; inappropriate affect; impaired problem solving; social withdrawal; behavior changes; signs of meningitis or other CNS disease; signs of self-neglect; sensory-perceptual deficits

Outcome Criteria:

Reduced disturbance in thought processes; increased orientation to reality

Interventions	Rationales
Assess and monitor mental and neurologic status: level of consciousness, orientation, memory, judgement, intellectual functioning, thought processes (flow and content), perception, and levels of anxiety, fear, and hopelessness; pre-existing mental illness	Establishes baseline; enhances ability to recognize problems early in order to initiate appropriate therapy and safety measures

Interventions	Rationales	Interventions	Rationales
Monitor for problems related to development of Altered Thought Processes, especially infection, electrolyte imbalance, dehydration, sensory-perceptual deficit, depression, hypoxemia, drug reactions; initiate appropriate interventions as needed; also see Hyperthermia, Fluid Volume Deficit, Risk for Infection, Altered Nutrition: Less than Body Requirements, Altered Bowel Elimination: Diarrhea, Altered Respiratory Function, Sleep Pattern Disturbance, Pain, Sensory-Perceptual Alteration (above), and Anxiety, Fatigue, Fear, Hopelessness, Powerlessness, Body Image Disturbance, Self-Esteem Disturbance, Grieving, Impaired Social Interaction, Social Isolation, Altered Sexuality Patterns, Ineffective Individual Coping, Ineffective Denial, Spiritual Distress (below)	Allows early recognition of problems related to cognitive impairment; encourages early interventions that may reverse cognition problems and dementia symptoms; promotes client safety, independence, and self-esteem	Refer to psychiatric services for work up, diagnosis, and treatment	Assists with determination of cause and early intervention; ART may help with dementia symptoms; other psychoactive drugs may provide some relief of symptoms
		Encourage involvement in self-care	Reorients to situation; promotes independence and self-esteem
		Teach memory enhancing and orientation techniques: use of a notebook or calendar to remember appointments and to make notes about symptoms, treatments, or questions for care providers; post daily schedules in an accessible location; keep personally significant pictures and objects at close hand; encourage interactions with family, significant others, and pets	Assists with compensation for memory losses

Interventions	Rationales	Interventions	Rationales
Promote consistent environment, routines, and caregivers as much as possible; introduce new caregivers gradually and only when absolutely necessary; decrease stimulation in the environment; limit choices that the client needs to make; provide simple directions, give one direction at a time, and allow appropriate time for client to grasp meaning and follow through on instruction	Assists with confusion management	Provide safe environment in the following ways: assess client for suicidal/self-abusive intentions; assess for hallucinations or delusions; provide a calm and caring presence that communicates concern; maintain as much client freedom as possible while insuring a safe environment; use restraints carefully to prevent injury, never in place of appropriate staff support, and never as punishment; be alert to increasing agitation and provide for seclusion or restraints as needed to prevent harm to self or others; manage "wandering" and confusion with constant surveillance by staff or significant others	Minimizes risks to client that can occur when thought processes are altered

Interventions	Rationales
Provide respite for family members and significant others who provide care during periods of dementia and confusion; encourage verbalizations about problems and concerns when providing care; assist in contact with support groups or individuals who provide one-on-one support; provide contact with home care and home-maker services so that clients in the community can receive care while significant others rest or socialize	Allows caregivers to "regroup" and restore energy levels that are required to provide the high levels of constant care required for clients with this problem; reconnects caregivers with social support systems

Evaluation:

The client:

1. Remains safe without physical injury
2. Experiences the least possible effects of altered thought processes with minimal disorientation, confusion, anxiety, or other dementia symptoms
3. Remains oriented to the environment and situation
4. Maintains the highest possible level of independence

Anxiety

A state in which the client experiences a vague, uneasy feeling in response to a non-specific or unknown threat.

Related to:

Symptom development; variability in the course of the disease; development of opportunistic diseases; knowledge deficits related to symptoms, opportunistic diseases, or potential treatments; threats to self-concept including changes in status or position at work or in family; loss of valued possessions; development of ethical dilemmas; actual, perceived, or feared loss of significant others; actual or anticipated changes in living environment including needs for hospitalization or home care; changes in socioeconomic situation related to decreasing ability to work; stigma; social isolation; unmet needs for security and independence; transmission of anxiety from significant others; lack of control

Defining Characteristics:

Stress manifested in physical, emotional, and cognitive symptoms

- **Subjective Findings:** Expresses fear, anger, denial, hostility, regret, helplessness, inability to sleep, concern over forgetfulness; makes statements about lack of self-confidence in abilities; verbalizes expectations of the worst possible outcomes; reports apprehension, worry, nervousness, loneliness, concerns about future
- **Objective Findings:** Physiologic symptoms of stress, insomnia, fatigue, apprehension; helplessness; nervousness; tension; fear; irritability; anger; withdrawal; lack of initiative; decreased attention span; difficulty learning/remembering; decreased coping ability; avoidance mechanisms; decreased communication abilities; unrealistic expectations

Outcome Criteria:

Anxiety decreased to manageable levels

Interventions	Rationales
Initiate interventions described in Anxiety in Secondary Prevention	Provides assessment and interventions for anxiety
Develop an atmosphere of mutual acceptance and trust: provide consistency in care and interpersonal interactions; use touch as appropriate; engage in honest communications around a variety of topics that are acceptable to the client; encourage hope, but avoid false reassurances; use open-ended questions and statements to encourage client to discuss anxieties; provide accurate and consistent information about prognosis and treatment	Establishes trust; promotes relaxation; provides necessary information for decision making; establishes a caring confidant who is willing to discuss a number of problematic issues; decreases feelings of loneliness and isolation

Interventions	Rationales
Encourage client interactions with family, significant others, and support systems	Decreases loneliness; assists with development of long-term support system; encourages honest discussions with individuals who can provide positive regard; allows initiation of problem-solving efforts
Address real life underlying problems that contribute to anxiety	Assists in determining sources of anxiety that may lead to interventions

Evaluation:

The client:

1. Discusses concerns
2. Uses effective coping strategies to manage anxiety
3. Verbalizes a decrease in anxiety

Fatigue

A state in which the client feels an overwhelming and sustained sense of exhaustion and decreased ability to maintain usual levels of physical or mental effort.

*Author's Note:

Fatigue is a common and frustrating symptom of HIV infection that generally worsens as HIV disease progresses.

Related to:

Infection with HIV and other opportunistic organisms; opportunistic cancers; fever; weakness; neuromuscular changes; anemia;

malnutrition; diarrhea; prolonged immobility; electrolyte imbalance; side effects of treatments (pharmacologic or radiation); overwhelming emotional demands; depression; anxiety and stress; insomnia; lack of social support; drug use; drug withdrawal; grief

Defining Characteristics:

Overwhelming and persistent feelings of tiredness

- **Subjective Findings:** Reports exhaustion after minimal activity; complains about shortness of breath, lack of energy, weakness, insomnia; discusses concerns about increasing physical problems; discusses lack of interest in usual relationships/ activities; complains about decreased libido; feels guilty about inability to keep up with responsibilities and usual activities

- **Objective Findings:** Dyspnea on mild exertion; requires frequent rest periods; inability to maintain usual activities; irritability; decreased ability to concentrate; lethargy; listlessness

Outcome Criteria:

Preservation and efficient use of energy

Interventions/Rationales

Initiate interventions described in Fatigue in Secondary Prevention; also refer to the following diagnoses which discuss interventions for related factors: Hyperthermia, Fluid Volume Deficit, Risk for Infection, Altered Nutrition: Less than Body Requirements, Altered Bowel Elimination: Diarrhea, Activity Intolerance, Altered Respiratory Function, Sleep Pattern Disturbance, Pain, Anxiety (above), and Fear, Hopelessness, Powerlessness, Grieving, Social Isolation, Ineffective Individual Coping, Spiritual Distress (below)

Evaluation:

The client:

1. Identifies causes of, or contributors to, fatigue
2. Establishes priorities for daily activities
3. Develops and follows a schedule that assures a balance of rest and physical activity

Fear

A state in which the client experiences a feeling of dread related to HIV infection, the anticipated chronic disease process, and/or the high morbidity and mortality associated with HIV disease.

Related to:

Progression of symptoms of chronic HIV disease; development of opportunistic diseases; development of complications such as sensory impairment, physical disabilities, weight loss, cognitive impairment, pain; the prospect of long-term disability and early death; need for hospitalization, home care, invasive procedures, medications, or radiation; loss or change in usual surroundings including significant others; lack of knowledge about disease process and treatment options

Defining Characteristics:

Feelings of dread or apprehension

- **Subjective Findings:** Describes fearful situations; discusses worries about real and anticipated losses; reports panic attacks or obsessions; verbalizes concerns about periods of dizziness, problems with sleeping, inability to concentrate, irritability, nightmares

- **Objective Findings:** Avoidance behaviors; attention, performance, or control deficits; behavioral manifestations of fear including crying, aggressive behaviors, hypervigilance, dysfunctional immobility, compulsive mannerisms, increased questioning; physical signs of fear including trembling, muscle tension, palpitations, tachycardia, increased blood pressure, shortness of breath, tachypnea, nausea and vomiting, anorexia, diarrhea, dry mouth, diaphoresis, dilated pupils; social paralysis; anger; grief

Outcome Criteria:

Fear reduced to a manageable level

Interventions/Rationales

Initiate interventions described in Fear in Secondary Prevention.

Evaluation:

The client:

1. Identifies personally acceptable coping mechanisms
2. Demonstrates ability to use coping mechanisms to manage fear levels
3. Verbalizes decreased levels of fear

Hopelessness

A state in which the individual sees limited or no alternatives or personal choices available and is unable to mobilize energy on own behalf.

*Author's Note:

Despite major recent treatment advances, HIV is still viewed by some as a hopeless situation, especially when symptoms develop and the client begins to experience deficits.

Related to:

Progression of HIV disease; poor response to ART; failing or deteriorating physical condition; impaired body image; new and unexpected signs and symptoms; pain and discomfort; fatigue; impaired functions; prolonged treatments with no positive results; painful or uncomfortable therapies; prolonged diagnostic studies with no results; social isolation; dependence; inability to achieve valued goals; loss or impairment of valued personal relationships; stress; loss of valued objects, activities, or pets; long-term stress; loss of spiritual belief system; prolonged activity restrictions

Defining Characteristics:

Apathy

- **Subjective Findings:** Expresses profound, overwhelming apathy in response to HIV that is perceived as an impossible situation with no solutions, "I might as well give up"; feels "empty, drained"; discusses lack of ambition, interest, initiative; feels vulnerable and helpless; refuses to participate in care

- **Objective Findings:** Slowed responses; lack of energy; poor or no response to ART; increased or decreased sleep; flat affect; decreased ability to solve problems and make decisions; unable to recognize solutions or sources of hope; anorexia and weight loss; severe depression; social withdrawal; anger; negative thought processes; confusion; poor communication skills; unrealistic perceptions; pessimism; suicidal ideation; frequent sighing

Outcome Criteria:

Realistic goal setting

Interventions/Rationales

Initiate interventions described in Hopelessness in Secondary Prevention.

Evaluation:

The client:

1. Reconsiders personal life values
2. Reinforces positive relationships with significant others
3. Sets realistic goals
4. Feels comfortable discussing a wide range of feelings and concerns including suicidal ideation

Powerlessness

A state in which the client perceives a lack of personal control over advancing HIV disease; a perception that one's actions will not significantly affect the outcome.

Related to:

Progressing HIV disease; lack of knowledge; poor response to ART; limited treatment options; expectations that HIV causes inevitable, uncontrollable consequences; feelings of doom; control perceived as a highly valued aspect of personal life; history of helplessness or dependence on others; perceived lack of control over health and health care decisions

Defining Characteristics:

Perceived lack of power

- **Subjective Findings:** Expresses discomfort or hostility over inability to control situation; discusses perceived lack of control over outcome; expresses dissatisfaction and frustration; discusses fears related to loss of abilities, control, or self-concept associated with HIV; verbalizes control issues related to health, health care, or future; reports anger, apathy, or passivity; refuses to participate in care or make decisions

- **Objective Findings:** Develops behaviors and attitudes that indicate dissatisfaction with lack of power: apathy, aggression, acting-out behaviors, anxiety, depression, resignation; increases dependence on others; becomes nonadherent to health care regimen

Outcome Criteria:

Exerts appropriate control

Interventions	Rationales
Initiate interventions described in Powerlessness in Secondary Prevention	Provides assistance focused on revealing areas where power and control can be maintained
Encourage client in activities that enhance personal control such as decision making related to type, amount, timing of health care; offering access to alternative health care practices; reinforcing activities and strengths that demonstrate client control; assisting client to make realistic future plans; discussing life planning related to legal issues such as wills, guardianship for children, financial plans, living wills, powers of attorney, and/or funeral plans	Enhances feelings of power; demonstrates ability to control issues even toward the end of life; reinforces self-worth

Evaluation:

The client:

1. Identifies control issues that are stressful
2. Realistically assesses factors that can be self-controlled
3. Makes and follows through on decisions

Body Image Disturbance

A state in which there is a disruption in the way an individual perceives her or his body image.

Related to:

Presence of lesions on skin or oral mucous membranes caused by KS, herpes simplex, herpes zoster, candida, staphylococcus, etc.; wasting syndrome; motor dysfunction; side effects of chemotherapy, radiation therapy, or ART; social stigmatization; social isolation; depression; chronic infection; decreasing control over body functions; pain; immobility; cultural and psychosocial influences that value youth, beauty, and strength; signs of aging (especially in younger clients) such as wrinkling, graying, hair loss, tooth loss, hearing and vision losses; lack of ability to accept changes in body structure or function; rigid ideas about appearance

Defining Characteristics:

Negative response to body changes caused by advancing HIV disease

- **Subjective Findings:** Expresses concerns about appearance; verbalizes feelings of shame, embarrassment, guilt, or revulsion related to changes in body structure and/or function; makes negative statements about body; expresses feelings of helplessness, hopelessness, powerlessness, and vulnerability; reports feeling useless and burdensome; discusses unrealistic ideas such as "Everything would be all right if I could just get rid of this KS lesion on my nose" or "No one can love a wrinkled woman who has diarrhea all the time"; refuses to interact in social situations or participate in care; expresses fears of rejection

- **Objective Findings:** Decrease in social interaction and communication skills; dresses to hide body changes; preoccupied with changes or losses; withdrawal; depression; nonassertive behaviors; fails to provide physical or grooming care for self; grief responses

Outcome Criteria:

Demonstrates increased acceptance of body image and self

Interventions	Rationales	Interventions	Rationales
Assess body image and self-concept; assist client to discuss changes caused by HIV infection; encourage client to express feelings about personal views of self and abilities; identify significance of client's culture, religion, race, sex, sexual orientation, and age on body image; monitor frequency of self-criticism; monitor client statements for information about body perception; determine client's and family's perceptions of body image as compared to reality; determine if body image changes have contributed to social isolation; determine client's personal meanings attached to changes in appearance or function; observe for preoccupation with appearance and client use of practices to change, improve, or hide problems with body structure or function	Establishes baseline and need for intervention; guides intervention	Create a relationship that is accepting; encourage honest discussion of problems related to body changes; avoid criticism of client concerns, comparisons with other clients who are worse off, or statements that devalue client concerns; provide information and reinforce previous information; clarify misconceptions	Establishes trust; demonstrates acceptance; validates client feelings; increases willingness to discuss difficult issues; encourages client to express feelings and thoughts; decreases knowledge deficits
		Acknowledge presence of changes; spend time with client; help client identify personal strengths; remind client of accomplishments; help client separate physical appearance from feelings of personal worth	Provides reality focus; reinforces positive aspects and base for working through body image issues

Interventions	Rationales	Interventions	Rationales
Assist client, as appropriate, to reduce impact of disfigurement in the following ways: use clothes, wigs, or cosmetics to cover or minimize problems; identify actions that can enhance appearance; encourage participation in support groups; facilitate increased social interactions; help client develop skills and abilities in alternate areas; support increased independence	Promotes positive self-image, independence, and self-esteem; facilitates decision making	Initiate interventions described in Decisional Conflict, Anxiety, Fear, Hopelessness, Powerlessness (above), and Self-Esteem Disturbance, Grieving, Social Isolation, Altered Sexuality Patterns, Ineffective Individual Coping, Ineffective Denial, Spiritual Distress (below) as needed	Body image disturbances affect, and are affected by, other problems identified in these nursing diagnoses
With client's approval, involve family and significant others in processes that enhance client's self-image: teach others about changes in body, expectations for further changes, potential therapies, and practical interventions; encourage others to accept client despite changes; describe expected psychosocial reactions to changes	Maintains important relationships with others; reinforces commitment and support; demonstrates unconditional acceptance; provides important emotional resource; allays fears	Encourage client to acknowledge realities of body changes: facilitate and reinforce client efforts to deal with changes; provide contacts with others who have dealt with similar changes; provide information on potential referrals to mental health and emotional support services and assist in establishing contact with resources that are appealing to the client; acknowledge all steps, no matter how small, toward acceptance and establishing personal control over life despite changes	Facilitates movements toward acceptance and adjustment; promotes independence and self-esteem

Evaluation:

The client:

1. Discusses feelings and expresses grief over losses
2. Develops methods for coping with changes
3. Continues to interact in important social relationships
4. Expresses more positive feelings about body image
5. Integrates HIV-related body changes into a total self-image that is personally acceptable

Self-Esteem Disturbance

A state of negative self-evaluation about self or personal capability.

Related to:

HIV-related changes in appearance or function; depression; pain; need for hospitalization or home care; loss of job or ability to work; death of significant other(s); weight loss; financial problems; relationship problems; loss of relationship(s); loss of control; multiple losses; ineffective relationships with parents/parental rejection; history of abusive relationships; unrealistic expectations of self; abuse of drugs or alcohol by self or family; co-dependency issues; legal difficulties; negative social or cultural influences that discriminate according to diagnosis of HIV, gender, race, age, or sexual orientation; inability to adjust to losses; cognitive-perceptual problems; inadequate knowledge or problem-solving ability; inadequate social support; loss of spiritual base; parenting failure

Defining Characteristics:

Poor self-image

- **Subjective Findings:** Verbalizes feelings of guilt or shame; evaluates self as incapable, inferior, or inadequate; denies problems; discusses feelings of lack of power or control; evaluates self as incapable of dealing with situation; discusses feelings of despair, guilt, inferiority, failure, defeat, frustration, unworthiness, hopelessness, powerlessness, helplessness, disappointment, worthlessness, isolation, depression, resentment

- **Objective Findings:** Self-negating behaviors; indecisiveness; inability to set goals or make decisions; poor problem-solving skills; signs of depression; self-abusive behaviors (including substance use, sexually acting-out behavior, and assuming the role of victim); projecting blame and responsibility to others; hesitancy to respond or initiate actions; poor eye contact; over-concern with somatic problems; unable to assume responsibility for self-care; distances self from significant other(s); withdrawal from activities and social interactions

Outcome Criteria:

Enhanced self-esteem

Interventions	Rationales	Interventions	Rationales
Establish a therapeutic relationship with the client: accept client's negative expressions without belittling, negating, teasing, or demeaning the client; express unconditional regard for the client despite negative statements; convey confidence in the client's abilities; provide genuine interest and concern; do not offer false praise; provide reliable and consistent information; clarify misconceptions; develop a safe environment for honest discussion of feelings and emotions; encourage client to explore personal values, develop assertive skills, practice verbalizing positive statements about self, and learn to accept and use positive criticism	Provides an environment in which the client can develop positive and realistic self-assessments; promotes ability to explore positive aspects about self; provides nonthreatening, supportive environment	Explore self-perception issues with client in a nonjudgmental manner: examine negative perceptions; analyze impact of others on self-esteem; discuss reasons for self-criticism or guilt; identify significance of issues (such as age, gender, sexual orientation, culture, chronic illness, religion, etc.) that influence self-esteem	Provides opportunities for understanding source of negative self-image; demonstrates acceptance of client despite litany of negative factors; reinforces self-worth
		Explore client's positive attributes and accomplishments: identify strengths, point out attractive features, reinforce past accomplishments especially related to parenting, job, and social arenas	Reinforces presence of positive attributes; enhances self-esteem

Interventions	Rationales	Interventions	Rationales
Recommend activities that show and reinforce personal capabilities: encourage realistic goal setting, increased responsibility, self-evaluation, and social interaction; encourage appropriate eye contact according to the client's culture when communicating with others; as health permits, encourage activities that contribute to or support others (such as volunteer work at community HIV organizations), increase social interactions (such as support groups or speaker's bureaus), and enhance physical capabilities (such as athletics or exercise)	Provides external source of esteem that may become internalized as successes accumulate; decreases self-absorption; provides interactions in which others can recognize client's worth and provide positive feedback	Teach appropriate interaction techniques to significant others such as assisting with identification of behaviors and verbalizations that negate client worth; discussing ways in which these actions can be moderated or eliminated; referring for professional family counseling as needed	Encourages support from meaningful others in the client's environment; may help to identify long-standing problems within the family or relationship; supports others' efforts to interact positively with client
		Identify underlying cause and initiate appropriate treatment or referrals	Some deep-seated causes of low self-esteem such as physical or sexual abuse, drug use, parental neglect, or overt discrimination require specialized treatment and counseling

Interventions	Rationales
Initiate interventions discussed in Ineffective Management of Therapeutic Regimen, Activity Intolerance, Instrumental Self-Care Deficit, Pain, Decisional Conflict, Anxiety, Fear, Hopelessness, Powerlessness, Body Image Disturbance (above), and Altered Family Processes, Grieving, Impaired Social Interaction, Social Isolation, Altered Sexuality Patterns, Ineffective Individual Coping, Ineffective Denial, Ineffective Family Coping, Risk for Violence: Self-Directed, Spiritual Distress (below) as appropriate	Problems identified in these nursing diagnoses contribute to or become a result of Self-Esteem Disturbance

Evaluation:

The client:

1. Realistically analyzes personal capabilities
2. Reflects on positive personal attributes
3. Develops and implements plans to deal with self-esteem problems
4. Verbalizes a more positive assessment of self

Situational Low Self-Esteem

A state of negative self-evaluation that develops in response to advancing HIV disease in a person who had a positive self-image prior to disease progression.

Related to:

Progression of HIV disease; poor response to ART; development of opportunistic diseases; loss of relationships; loss of ability to continue education or work goals; negative social or cultural definitions of HIV and AIDS; multiple losses (actual, anticipated, or perceived); financial problems; need for hospitalization or home care; change in living conditions; grief; discrimination based on diagnosis; loss of parenting role

Defining Characteristics:

Negative changes in self-image due to HIV infection

- **Subjective Findings:** Expresses feelings of guilt, worthlessness or shame; evaluates self as incapable, inadequate, or inferior because of HIV infection or lack of response to ART; feels powerless, hopeless, or helpless; expects social discrimination because of HIV infection

- **Objective Findings:** Self-negating behaviors; indecisiveness; inability to set goals or make decisions; poor problem-solving skills; signs of depression; self-abusive behaviors (including substance use, sexually acting-out behavior, and assuming the role of victim); denial of problems; projecting blame and responsibility to others; self-neglect; social isolation

Outcome Criteria:

Enhanced self-esteem

Interventions	Rationales
Explore self-perception issues with client: examine negative perceptions, discuss reasons for self-criticism or guilt, identify significance of HIV disease progression as it influences self-esteem	Provides opportunities for understanding source of negative self-image; demonstrates acceptance of client despite HIV disease; reinforces self-worth
Initiate interventions discussed in Self-Esteem Disturbance (above)	Provides assessment and intervention for general self-esteem problems
Facilitate client interactions with others who have dealt with HIV infection: contact HIV service organizations to determine types of services available (many provide one-on-one encounters, support groups, and educational and volunteer opportunities)	Shows client that s/he is not alone in having to deal with these issues; provides role models who have worked through problems associated with HIV disease progression; provides opportunities for esteem-enhancing activities among non-judgmental peers
If problems persist, initiate appropriate referrals	Situational low self-esteem may progress to chronic low self-esteem if precipitating factor is allowed to become the overriding concern in the client's life

Evaluation:

The client:

1. Discusses self-perceptions and capabilities realistically
2. Reflects on positive personal attributes
3. Reassesses impact of HIV disease on self-evaluation
4. Develops strategies and support structures that enhance self-esteem

Altered Family Processes

A state in which a family that normally functions effectively experiences a challenge to its functional status when a family member is faced with advancing HIV disease.

*Author's Note:

As HIV disease progresses, the family will often become more involved with health care and support. This is true even in families that were not able to accept the client and the disease initially. At this point, the client may move back home, either into a relative's home or at least to a nearby location, thus increasing the family's interactions and responsibilities. These activities add stress to the function of the family even if there is a well-established, loving relationship with the client. All families who are dealing with HIV disease need extra support and assistance. Remember that "family" is defined by the client. The family may be made up of blood relatives, friends, or significant others who may or may not be sexual partners. Families with dependent children will have additional concerns about continuing child care as adult(s) become ill and concerns about long-term issues related to guardianship and support in the event of the adult(s)' death.

Related to:

Progression of HIV disease; observation of a family member who is dealing with pain, discomfort, and deterioration; expensive and time-consuming treatments; disruption of family routines; change in family member's ability to function in established, comfortable manner; financial burdens on the family related to health care requirements and changes in employment or income; emotional changes as family member with HIV disease becomes more dependent; blame; guilt; fear; anger; changes in living situation; changes in roles of family members; grief and anticipatory grieving

Defining Characteristics:

Family system does not adapt to changes

- **Subjective Findings:** *Client* complains that family is not being supportive; discusses loss of intimacy with family members and feelings of being outcast; blames self for all familial problems; feels family does not provide respect, support, or care; *Family Member(s)* express feelings of anger, guilt, shame, rejection, fatigue, fear, anxiety, grief; discuss concerns about ability to continue support for client

- **Objective Findings:** Poor communication within family; physical, emotional, spiritual, or safety needs of individual not met by family; financial stressors; inability to adapt to health care requirements, especially hospitalization and home health care; inappropriate level and direction of energy; inability to accept appropriate assistance; rigidity in roles and functions without demonstration of ability to adapt as HIV disease progresses; lack of involvement in community activities

Outcome Criteria:

Maintenance of supportive family structure

Interventions	Rationales
Encourage family to discuss issues that develop as HIV disease progresses; encourage family members to express concerns, fears, positive and negative feelings about the situation; assess family strengths; list basic problems realistically; discover problems that are based on inadequate information related to disease progression, treatment options, community support, etc.	Initiates discussion of difficult issues; identifies knowledge deficits
Establish trusting relationship with family members: allow confidential and supportive communications that encourage family members to discuss difficult issues; provide consistent and accurate information; encourage continued participation in client care; provide support and education as needed	Promotes feelings of confidence in nurse as a trustworthy support; encourages disclosure of feelings and concerns that can lead to nursing interventions; supports family members in their efforts to support each other

Interventions	Rationales	Interventions	Rationales
Teach family members basic information about HIV disease: expectations related to disease progression, treatment options, and resources	Allays anxiety and fear; provides basis for realistic planning	Assist family to resolve identified problems: encourage expressions of guilt, hostility, and anger; involve family members in care as they are able; include family members in caregiving decisions; teach caregiving procedures; reinforce use of appropriate safety measures; encourage respite periods; provide information about community resources for home care, nutritional assistance, transportation, financial support, emotional support, etc; provide anticipatory guidance as disease progresses (assist with increasing home care needs, prepare for losses, discuss future plans, assist in discussion of end of life issues, etc.); refer to family therapy as appropriate	Facilitates interactions that can lead to positive change; defuses potentially volatile situations; decreases knowledge deficits related to care giving and support services; prevents caregiver burnout
Assess ability of the family to provide needed support: Will assistance be offered to client in a loving and supportive manner or is care seen as an unwelcome obligation? Are housing facilities appropriate for the safe care of the client? Will financial problems develop as the disease progresses? Is fear of infection a concern for family members? Is fear of discrimination a concern? Will the primary caregiver(s) be supported and provided with respite care?	Provides basis for intervention recommendations		

Interventions	Rationales
Provide continuing support to individual within family who has HIV infection	When family problems are overwhelming, sometimes the best solution is to help client find alternative sources of support (at least until family members are better able to accept the client and the disease process)
Assist client to plan for appropriate child care under a variety of circumstances; encourage the development of a will with guardianship provisions	Provides assurances that children will receive care according to client desires

Evaluation:

Family members:

1. Verbalize concerns about ability to provide care
2. Communicate concerns to other family members
3. Resolve issues
4. Maintain support system for all family members

Grieving

A state in which the client experiences a natural human response to an actual or perceived loss.

*Author's Note:

Loss characterizes HIV disease, providing the need for major support during grief processes. As HIV disease progresses, infected individuals will potentially experience losses in all aspects of their physical, social, emotional, and professional lives. In addition, many HIV-infected individuals have experienced the loss of significant others through death or abandonment. All of these losses present the need for active grief support. The significant others of HIV-infected clients will also need assistance with their own grief work as they watch the deterioration process in their loved one.

Related to:

Multiple losses related to the progression of HIV disease including loss of health, appearance, body function, capability to perform usual activities, job, career, family, friends, partners, pets, housing, personal objects, social and economic status, health insurance, hopes, dreams, independence; presence of a potentially terminal disease; lifestyle changes; lack of a social support system; stigma and discrimination related to HIV disease, sexual orientation, and/or drug use; lack of response to ART

Defining Characteristics:

Physical and psychosocial reactions to loss

- **Subjective Findings:** Reports loss(es) that are personally meaningful and significant; verbalizes feelings of guilt, anger, denial, despair, worthlessness, sorrow, anxiety, self-blame, loneliness, fatigue, helplessness, shock, yearning, numbness; describes suicidal ideation

- **Objective Findings:** Depressed affect; decreased ability/desire to communicate with others; increased time in bed; increased sleeping time; selling or giving away possessions; neglects personal grooming, nutrition, and personal care needs

Outcome Criteria:

Integration of loss(es) into life and discovery of meaning in illness and death

Interventions	Rationales
Assist client to discuss loss(es): help client identify (name) loss(es) that have been experienced; encourage discussions that help the client identify the personal meanings of each loss; allow client to express emotions and feelings about the loss(es); ask client about previous losses and previous coping methods; encourage discussion of fears related to each loss; allow for periods of silence and crying	Provides assessment information that will be used as a base to plan interventions; recognizes the importance of loss(es); establishes an open, trusting relationship in which frank discussions about loss and grief can occur; promotes self-reflection
Identify client's usual coping mechanisms; reinforce healthy mechanisms such as talking to friends, exercising, meditating, etc.; refer to counseling for unhealthy responses such as drinking, drugging, acting-out sexually or physically, withdrawal	Reinforces healthy responses that have a history of success; circumvents return to less healthy coping mechanisms

Interventions	Rationales
Explain grief reactions that frequently occur (shock, denial, disbelief, isolation, bargaining, depression, acceptance, physical responses); explain that each individual works through losses in a unique way and that the client and/or family will not necessarily progress in any set pattern	Establishes a knowledge base; allows client to progress without feeling the need to meet goals and stages
Provide support as client works through grief reaction; explain need for various reactions to family members and caregivers; discuss ways to support client during various phases of grief reaction with significant others; encourage support of significant others; promote grief work	Supports client with specific interventions at each phase of the grief reaction; supports family members who must cope with client's reactions while dealing with their own problems related to loss
Denial: do not push client to move past denial before s/he is emotionally capable; observe and prevent potentially dangerous activities that may occur as a result of denial (i.e., insisting on driving when vision is impaired)	

Interventions	Rationales	Interventions	Rationales

Isolation/Rejection of Others: allow privacy; explain need for solitude to significant others; encourage gradual increases in amount of social interaction

Depression: acknowledge grief and promote sharing of feelings about loss; assess level of depression and provide appropriate interventions related to suicide prevention and/or consultations with mental health professionals

Anger: encourage verbalizations about anger; support family and caregivers who may be the focus of anger; encourage identification of appropriate target for anger, and discuss issues important to specific problem; discuss ways to increase personal independence and control since these losses frequently cause anger reactions

Guilt: encourage discussions about feelings related to guilt; help client identify reality related to the loss (Was lack of knowledge involved? Were positive actions taken? Was lack of control an issue?); refrain from buying into client's system of "shoulds" and "should nots," return instead to a reality-based discussion (Maybe you should have, but could you have? Would it have been possible at that time and in those circumstances?)

Fear: maintain safe environment; assist with learning about ways to compensate for physical and sensory-perceptual losses; also see Activity Intolerance, Impaired Home Maintenance Management, Sensory-Perceptual Alteration (above)

Interventions	Rationales
Identify and refer to resources that will support grief work (mental health counselors, support groups, spiritual leaders, etc.); assist client and/or family members to establish contact with desired support systems	Provides long-term support for the grieving process

Evaluation:

The client:

1. Expresses grief and, in the process, discovers meanings of loss and coping methods
2. Begins to cope with losses
3. Maintains social contact with supportive significant others

Anticipatory Grieving

A state in which the client and/or significant others experience reactions in response to an expected significant loss.

Related to:

Progression of HIV disease; anticipated losses including those related to function, capability, income, possessions, independence, relationships, control, body image, self-respect, goal attainment, having children, watching children mature, support systems, spiritual base or dignity, as well as actual death

Defining Characteristics:

Expectations of loss

- **Subjective Findings:** Expresses distress related to potential losses; states that anticipated losses are personally significant; feels resigned to fate, anxious, lonely, tired; blames self; discusses hope for interventions that will prevent losses

- **Objective Findings:** Denial; anger; bargaining; guilt; sorrow; depression; change in social and communication patterns; social withdrawal; tearfulness; ambivalence; sleep and appetite disturbances; disinterest in or difficulty carrying out ADLs; hostility; irritability

Outcome Criteria:

Preparation for dealing with anticipated losses

Interventions	Rationales
Encourage client to identify losses that are anticipated	Assesses extent of anticipatory grief; provides information for use in interventions
Help client assess each anticipated loss in a realistic manner: ask client to describe personal meanings related to each potential loss; provide information about treatments and interventions that will help allay difficulties associated with physical and functional losses	Encourages client to initiate coping processes and plan for future potential losses; provides information that can decrease fears and concerns; promotes hope

Interventions	Rationales
Facilitate grieving for those losses that are imminent; see Grieving (above)	Acknowledges all losses; validates the importance of each loss; provides basis for closure and growth
Encourage client to share concerns with supportive individuals such as family, friends, counselors, religious/spiritual leaders, support group peers, etc.	Reinforces the importance of the support system; gives support individuals insight into client's problems; promotes cohesiveness with family/ significant others
Facilitate decision-making processes, see Decisional Conflict (above)	Encourages client to develop plans prior to losses; provides sense of accomplishment and control; relieves anxiety

Evaluation:

The client/significant other:

1. Discusses anticipated losses
2. Expresses grief
3. Develops plans for allaying, delaying, or coping with future losses
4. Shares concerns with significant others

Dysfunctional Grieving

A state in which the individual suffers a prolonged response to grief that is unresolved and detrimental.

Related to:

Multiple losses with unresolved grief; negation of loss by others; social isolation; assuming the role of "the strong one";

chronic mental or physical illness; inability to attend to grieving because of problems associated with dealing with HIV disease and related physical, psychosocial, and financial problems; fear of the mourning process

Defining Characteristics:

Prolonged or delayed reactions to loss

- **Subjective Findings:** Reports problems with concentration, developing new interests, low self-esteem, eating, sleeping, activity, and libido levels; discusses feelings of despair and hopelessness

- **Objective Findings:** Inhibition, suppression or absence of emotional reactions to loss; prolonged denial of loss; spends excessive time discussing past and reliving experiences; decreased participation in formerly helpful spiritual activities; hopelessness; suicidal ideation; somatic expressions of fear such as hyperventilation, choking, dyspnea; social isolation or withdrawal; fails to restructure life after loss

Outcome Criteria:

Progressive resolution of grief

Interventions	Rationales	Interventions	Rationales
Initiate interventions described in Grieving (above)	Prolonged grief reactions may have developed because the client did not receive appropriate and supportive interventions at the time of initial losses	Assist with identifying and developing interventions for problems that can increase, delay, or prolong grief; see also Ineffective Therapeutic Regimen, Noncompliance (Nonadherence), Activity Intolerance, Impaired Home Maintenance Management, Instrumental Self-Care Deficit, Sleep Pattern Disturbance, Pain, Sensory-Perceptual Disturbance, Altered Thought Process, Fatigue, Altered Family Process (above), and Impaired Social Interaction, Social Isolation, Altered Sexuality Patterns, Relocation Stress, Suicide, Spiritual Distress (below)	Numerous problems can impact on the grief process and must be considered as the client is assisted to complete grief work
Determine if client is "stuck" in a particular phase or with a particular emotional grief response; develop specific interventions to cope with these specific problems; also see Decisional Conflict, Anxiety, Fear, Hopelessness, Powerlessness (above), and Ineffective Individual Coping, Ineffective Denial (below)	Focuses interventions on identified area of need		

Interventions	Rationales
Help client acknowledge awareness of loss: provide opportunities to discuss loss; restate reality in nonthreatening manner; present factual information; do not argue with client or significant others about reality of loss; use guided imagery or role playing to allow client to confront loss	Promotes recognition of loss as meaningful to the client; initiates recognition of need to grieve
Promote adaptation to loss: facilitate contact with others who have experienced similar losses; encourage use of previously helpful (and healthy) coping mechanisms; provide consistent and correct information, clarify misconceptions, correct misinformation; offer hope for successful adaptation; encourage time for rest, relaxation, exercise, and nutrition; provide contacts with mental health professionals, religious/spiritual leaders, family, and friends who are acceptable supports for the client	Encourages positive activities that can move client through grief process; decreases knowledge deficits; acknowledges need for "time off" to replenish energy stores; promotes social interactions for support

Evaluation:

The client:

1. Acknowledges personally meaningful loss(es)
2. Initiates efforts to deal with loss(es)
3. Reports decreasing discomfort related to grief
4. Moves into grief work process

Parental Role Conflict

A state in which a parent experiences role conflict in response to his/her own advancing HIV infection.

*Author's Note:

HIV is a family disease. When one member becomes infected, the whole family is affected. Many HIV-infected individuals in the United States are parents. Some of their children were born prior to the parent's infection and are thus at risk of suffering the effects of the parent's illness and potential death. Other children were born to women who were already infected and may be infected themselves. (See Introduction for a discussion of the risk and refer to a pediatric text on HIV infection for the nursing care required in families with infected children.) The fathers of these children may also be ill and at risk of dying. In some families, the children may have already experienced the loss of one parent as a result of HIV infection and are now living through the process in which they may lose their remaining parent.

Related to:

Parent's advancing HIV infection; decreased parental role; multiple health care providers in the home; hospitalization of the parent; multiple family stressors; financial problems; inadequate social supports; single parents who provide sole support for children; disruption of family routines as parent experiences acute exacerbations and/or chronic deterioration; health care system that does not consider family cultural, social, and child-rearing norms

Defining Characteristics:

Children without parental support

- **Subjective Findings:** *Parent* expresses doubts about abilities to continue to care for child(ren); complains about loss of control and decision-making capabilities within family; identifies disruptions in family processes; verbalizes feelings of guilt, fear, anger, anxiety, frustration, or inadequacy in relation to child care

- **Objective Findings:** *Children* demonstrate poor nutrition and hygiene, lack of parental control in social and academic activities, and/or clinging behaviors, fear, anxiety, depression, guilt, anger; older children may have taken over parental roles, especially in a single-parent family; *Parent* displays evidence of stress, fear, anxiety, guilt, fatigue, depression, or anger

Outcome Criteria:

Family receives support required to maintain appropriate support of children

Interventions	Rationales
Assess needs of family in a home visit if possible: determine usual family routines, individual roles, and family member responsibilities; determine if these norms are being disrupted by the parent's illness	Provides baseline assessment and data for planning interventions
Minimize disruption of family routines as much as possible by encouraging creative actions to maintain family rituals (for example: provide family meals at the parent's bedside or encourage older children to visit parent's room at bedtime for storytelling or prayers); and by encouraging children to continue school and social activities	Encourages maintenance of family interactions and routines
Assist client to use assistive devices to maintain contact with children and adult family members while hospitalized (i.e., telephone calls, letters, video- or audio-taped messages, etc.)	Reminds children of their parent's concern even when the parent has to be away because of acute illness

Interventions	Rationales	Interventions	Rationales
Help family incorporate home health care into family routine: older children can assist in care; younger ones can be welcomed into the parent's room as appropriate; schedule care routines so as not to interrupt normal family rituals related to meals and bedtime	Maintains family contacts, helps children feel that they are an important part of the family	If family is demonstrating problems, assist with the identification of specific problems; explore family strengths and usual family coping mechanisms; discuss strategies for normalizing family life (taking into consideration cultural, social, and relationship norms of the family); assist family to determine best course of action; encourage use of existing support systems; facilitate entry into community support systems as needed	Allows family processes to continue as needs for changes and additional support are determined
If family continues to function in a supportive and functional manner, offer continuing support, education, and resource identification that will help to maintain family function	Establishes relationship that can be used in the event of family crisis		

Interventions	Rationales
Encourage parents to determine child care concerns for emergency situations and to develop plans that are legally binding: If parent becomes sick and has to go to the hospital, who will be available to care for children? If parent dies, who are the legal guardians for the children?; determine extent to which these issues have been discussed and assist in further planning as needed; encourage parents to draw up wills, powers of attorney, and financial arrangements for children early in the course of the disease; assist parent to share decision making with children who are old enough to understand	Decreases anxiety because parent knows that child(ren) will be cared for in the event of an acute problem or death; assists parent to maintain control and provide direction for child(ren) during illness or death; decreases anxiety for child(ren) who know what will happen if problems arise
Facilitate use of community support systems for children whose parent(s) have HIV infection such as counseling, support groups, etc.	Assists child(ren) to adjust to conditions; provides support for long-term issues related to loss of a parent, guilt, grief, and disrupted childhood

Evaluation:

The parent(s):

1. Continues to provide support for children
2. Identifies and takes steps to plan for and/or rectify problems
3. Verbalizes decreased stress and anxiety related to providing long-term support for children

The child(ren):

1. Identifies resources and sources of support for times of crisis
2. Maintains a positive relationship with the parent
3. Demonstrates decreasing levels of anxiety, fear, anger, and/or acting-out behaviors
4. Adjusts to alternative care from designated guardians or foster care

Impaired Social Interaction

A state in which an individual experiences negative, insufficient, or unsatisfactory responses from social interactions.

Related to:

Advancing HIV disease; chronic, potentially fatal disease; loss of body function; hearing or visual deficits; lack of motivation; fatigue; severe anxiety; dependent behavior; hopelessness; powerlessness; lack of self-care skills; poor impulse control; depression; egocentric behaviors; language, cultural, religious, economic, environmental, geographic barriers; social isolation; substance use; loss of spouse/partner through death or desertion; need for hospitalization or home care; lack of social skills; loss of ability to work; limited physical mobility; self-concept disturbance; altered thought processes; lack of available significant others/friends; communication barriers

Defining Characteristics:

Lack of stable, supportive relationships

- **Subjective Findings:** Verbalizes discomfort in social situations; reports unsatisfactory interactions with family and peers; discusses need for support from others; acknowledges that established relationships are superficial; blames others for interpersonal problems; reports feelings of anxiety in social interactions; discusses feelings of incompetency in social interactions

- **Objective Findings:** *Client* unable to receive or communicate a sense of belonging, caring, or interest in others; uses unsuccessful or inappropriate social behaviors; unaware of how she or he is perceived by others; exhibits dependent behaviors; *Family* reports changes in interactions with client

Outcome Criteria:

Improved ability to relate to others

Interventions	Rationales
Assist with the development of a positive self-image: develop an individual and supportive relationship with the client; encourage client to explore relationship and interpersonal issues; help client list positive personal characteristics and strengths as well as social limitations; implement interactions discussed in Self-Esteem Disturbance, Situational Low Self-Esteem, Anxiety (above)	Develops a trusting relationship with the nurse in order for interventions to progress; helps client assess strengths as well as weaknesses; addresses poor self-concept that is a common underlying problem in impaired social interactions

Interventions	Rationales	Interventions	Rationales
Identify with the client issues that increase problems in social interactions; support healthy defenses; help client problem solve around specific issue	Allows mutual assessment of problems; encourages client to take responsibility for problem areas; see also Activity Intolerance, Instrumental Self-Care Deficit, Sleep Pattern Disturbance, Pain, Decisional Conflict, Sensory-Perceptual Alteration, Altered Thought Process, Fatigue, Fear, Hopelessness, Powerlessness, Altered Family Processes, Grief (above), and Altered Sexuality Patterns, Ineffective Individual Coping, Ineffective Denial, Ineffective Family Coping, Spiritual Distress (below)	Allow client to practice alternative or new behaviors in a safe environment: set up role play experiences based on client-identified situations; encourage client to take on the role of the other in some of these role plays; provide honest and supportive feedback, pointing out successes and asking for ways to alter less successful interactions; reinforce client attitude of respect for the rights and perspective of others; discuss possibility of client involvement in transactional analysis classes or support groups	Provides experiential learning that is most appropriate for skill development; allows critique and immediate experimentation with alternative interactions; encourages client to see interactions from the other's perspective; enhances feelings of capability and self-control in social situations

Interventions	Rationales
Encourage expanded use of skills in "real" social situations such as in established relationships, in developing new relationships, in support groups, or in groups of people with similar interests or concerns; debrief client on how interactions felt, discuss alternative ways of interacting in these situations and role play revised situations	Allows generalization of skills learned in a controlled environment; provides continuing support, learning, and skill development
Provide supportive feedback and encouragement; give positive feedback in situations where client initiates social interactions, expands areas of interest and interaction, and/or makes informed decisions	Rewards client for taking initiative; points out positive interactions; helps client gain confidence and independence
Refer to community support systems as appropriate: HIV service organizations, mental health and family counseling, social services	Provides continuing support; assists client to cope with problems related to impaired social interactions

Evaluation:

The client:

1. Acknowledges personal strengths and limitations in social interactions
2. Develops new behaviors and interaction skills
3. Develops self-confidence in using skills to improve established relationships and develop new relationships
4. Verbalizes decreased anxiety in social situations and satisfaction with social relationships

Social Isolation

A state in which the client and/or family experiences aloneness that is perceived to be negative or threatening and to have been imposed by others.

Related to:

Stigma associated with HIV infection, sexual orientation, and/or substance use; social fears related to communicable nature of HIV infection; family rejection; withdrawal from people and activities; advancing HIV disease; sensory-perceptual deficits; altered thought processes; physical disfigurement; extreme anxiety; depression; loss of significant other(s) through death or abandonment; poverty; need for hospitalization or home health care; substance use; loss of means of transportation; loss of job/career; alienation; low self-esteem; language problems; geographic distance from family; impaired mobility; body image disturbance; inadequate personal resources; unaccepted social behavior

Defining Characteristics:

Isolation from society

- **Subjective Findings:** Expresses feelings of loneliness, isolation, uselessness, hopelessness, depression, lack of purpose in life, rejection; states perception that isolation has been imposed by others; verbalizes desire for more human contact; reports multiple losses, barriers to social contact, changes in living arrangements or inadequate social support system; acknowledges inability to concentrate and make decisions; describes changes in sleeping or eating patterns; discusses insecurity in social situations

- **Objective Findings:** Inability to make decisions or delays decision making; increasing evidence of physical or mental deterioration; depression, anxiety, or anger; failure to interact with others; aggressive or hostile behaviors; absence of supportive others, lack of visitors; withdrawal; inability or refusal to communicate

Outcome Criteria:

Maintenance of social relationships or adaptation to changes in relationships

Interventions	Rationales
Assess client perceptions of causes of loneliness: encourage discussions about aloneness; use active listening; ask open-ended questions that focus on isolation; restate client responses and ask for clarification; help client validate feelings	Initiates therapeutic relationship; assesses causes of isolation; provides base for development of specific interventions
Assist with developing plans to deal with specifically identified problems: determine transportation alternatives and provide resources; assist with aesthetic problems (demonstrate use of make up to hide lesions, promote dental care to improve oral hygiene, use clothing to hide wasting or wigs to cover hair loss, etc.); use appropriate interventions as described in Activity Intolerance, Instrumental Self-Care Deficit, Sleep Pattern Disturbance, Pain, Sensory-Perceptual Alteration, Altered Thought Process, Anxiety, Fatigue, Fear, Hopelessness, Powerlessness, Body Image Disturbance, Self-Esteem Disturbance, Altered Family Processes, Grieving, Impaired Social Interaction (above), and Caregiver Role Strain, Ineffective Individual Coping, Ineffective Family Coping, Spiritual Distress (below)	Provides interventions to deal with specific problems that may be contributing to social isolation

Interventions	Rationales
With client's permission, encourage interactions with significant others: instruct significant others in mechanisms of HIV transmission and prevention of transmission; involve them in providing care; encourage communications through letters and telephones; identify specific times when client is well-rested and not being subjected to treatments when visitors are welcomed	Supports continuing efforts of significant others to be involved in client's life; reassures others about risk of infection; provides positive environment for social interaction
Spend social time with client when treatments and physical care are not required: interact in a social nature by discussing topics of interest that are not necessarily related to HIV disease; use touch as acceptable to the client; avoid using protective equipment such as masks and gloves unless there is a risk of blood exposure	Expresses unconditional regard for client that extends beyond providing physical care; models social interaction skills; provides human contact

Interventions	Rationales
Assist client to develop plans for expanding social interactions: identify activities that interest the client; provide resources for social interaction in the community (volunteer work, speaking engagements, working at local HIV service organizations, day care centers, support groups, initiating telephone contact with significant others, etc.); promote realistic course of action that does not overburden the client; encourage risk taking, help client identify potential barriers to social contacts and develop means to overcome the barriers; support client during progress to develop arena for social interactions; see also Decisional Conflict (above)	Promotes independence and decision making, provides opportunities to increase social interactions; encourages planning to circumvent barriers prior to their development

Evaluation:

The client:

1. Receives social support as needed
2. Is involved in activities that increase social interactions
3. Adjusts to losses that inhibit social interaction

Altered Sexuality Patterns

A state in which an individual or partner expresses concerns about the client's sexuality as it is or will be affected by HIV.

*Author's Note:

Sexuality is a major aspect of human existence that continues despite the presence or progression of HIV disease. Many HIV-infected people will lose interest in sexual activity at this point for a variety of reasons. For some, abstinence is imposed by physical, social, and/or individual losses; for others, abstinence is chosen in order to prevent further transmissions, prevent pregnancy, or conserve energy. Clients who wish to maintain sexual interactions with others need to have appropriate information in order to make safe and healthy decisions. Remember that sexuality encompasses more than sexual intercourse. Sometimes the primary need is to have the feeling of attachment and personal touch that can only be provided by an emotionally attached significant sexual other.

Related to:

Progressing HIV disease; fatigue and lack of energy; pain; presence of chronic vaginal or anal infection(s); side effects of drug and/or radiation therapy; altered self-concept and/or body image disturbance; self-esteem problems; loss of sexual partner through death or abandonment; lack of privacy; presence of stressors related to

health care, finances, conflicts with religious or personal values; fear of transmitting or contracting HIV infection; fear of contracting other STDs; fear of rejection if disclosure of infection is made or if partner refuses to use protection; substance use; fear of failure; fear of pregnancy; depression; anxiety; guilt; negative social attitude toward sexual activity after HIV infection; lack of information about safety and alternative means of sexual expression; social isolation; decreased sex drive

Defining Characteristics:

Concern over the effect of an HIV diagnosis on sexual function

- **Subjective Findings:** Expresses concern about sexuality; identifies concern about involvement in sexual behaviors that place others at risk of HIV infection; discusses fears about changes in sexual function if risk reducing measures are instituted; verbalizes guilt, shame, or stigma; discusses frustrations related to sexuality; acknowledges change in sexual behavior or activities; expresses concerns about loss of appearance or function that could decrease ability to develop sexual relationships; discusses problems related to ability to develop or maintain an erection, inability to achieve orgasm, or pain during intercourse

- **Objective Findings:** Reluctance to discuss sexual issues; guilt; fear; shame; lack of interest in sexual issues

Outcome Criteria:

Sexual function as desired

Interventions	Rationales	Interventions	Rationales
Initiate interventions discussed in Altered Sexuality Patterns in Secondary Prevention	Continues support for education and skill development for maintenance of sexual intimacy	Assess for presence of contributing factors and initiate care as outlined in Risk for Infection, Risk for Infection Transmission, Activity Intolerance, Sleep Pattern Disturbance, Pain, Anxiety, Fatigue, Fear, Body Image Disturbance, Self-Esteem Disturbance, Grieving, Impaired Social Interaction, Social Isolation (above)	Provides care for specifically identified problems
Assess for concerns about sexual function: support sexual activity that is acceptable to the client and partner, that reduces risk, and that enhances feelings of personal worth; provide information and support for changes in sexual activities that are unsafe and/or detrimental to the emotional and physical security of the client; avoid personal judgements about client's means of sexual expression; reinforce need for touch and emotional closeness to another individual	Provides baseline assessment; determines need for intervention		

Evaluation:

The client:

1. Discusses concerns about sexuality
2. Verbalizes satisfaction with sexuality and intimacy issues

Caregiver Role Strain

A state in which a caregiver (other than a professional health care provider) experiences physical, emotional, economic, or social difficulty in performing the caregiver role.

*Author's Note:

Family caregiving is a common experience for HIV-infected clients. The uncertainty of disease progression and the chronic nature of the disease make home care a more acceptable alternative for many HIV-infected clients. Caregivers often include partners, spouses, and parents (especially mothers) of adult clients as well as children, siblings, in-laws, step parents, and friends. It is important to remember that HIV is a family disease and that more than one member of the family may be infected. Sometimes caregivers are dealing with their own infected status while they are caring for their significant others. This serves to increase the burden and stress.

Related to:

Advancing HIV disease in the care receiver, especially after an acute episode requiring hospitalization; increased care needs of the care receiver; substance use by either the care receiver or caregiver; co-dependency; conflicting role demands in the caregiver (i.e., career, child care, responsibilities to other members of the family, etc.); impaired health status of the caregiver; caregiver lack of experience in providing health care; history of familial dysfunction or poor caregiver-care receiver relationship prior to advancing HIV disease; caregiver lack of coping patterns; need for direct, long-term, 24 hour care in the home; unpredictable course of HIV disease; care receiver develops psychological, cognitive, sensory-perceptual problems; care receiver develops bizarre behaviors, becomes incontinent, or manifests signs of dementia; relative difficulty of required health care interventions; caregiver apprehension related to client's health and/or ability to provide care; caregiver experiences or anticipates multiple losses related to relationship with care receiver, career, finances, social system, etc.; caregiver feelings of depression, anxiety, anger, guilt; caregiver and/or care receiver have unrealistic expectations; caregiver experiences isolation as well as insufficient rest, relaxation, respite, finances

Defining Characteristics:

Decreased ability to provide home care

- **Subjective Findings:** Caregiver reports feeling exhausted; discusses declining health status; verbalizes feelings of depression, loss, grief, stress, anxiety, sleep pattern disturbances, poor self-concept; relates emotional response to changes in expected relationship (i.e., son is supposed to care for mother in her old age instead of her caring for him in a terminal disease, partner/spouse expected a sharing of life burdens, children want to depend on parent for support, etc.); discusses family/role conflicts related to caregiving role; describes withdrawal from social contacts and usual leisure activities due to fatigue, sense of responsibility, fear of stigma or discrimination

- **Objective Findings:** Caregiver unable to complete required tasks; declining health; emotional lability; social withdrawal; refuses to allow others to provide respite care; insists on providing 24 hour care; becomes preoccupied with caregiving routine; apprehensive; anxious; angry; depressed

Outcome Criteria:

Effective support for caregiver

Interventions	Rationales	Interventions	Rationales
Assess care needs and capabilities of the HIV-infected client: ability to perform ADLs, psychosocial status, cognitive status, and behavioral issues; prognosis; degree of impairment; intensity of required care; relationship with the caregiver; alternative support system; willingness to accept help, especially from designated caregiver	Provides baseline assessment that should be reassessed on a regular basis as client status changes; identifies areas of difficulty in provision of care	Assess care needs and capabilities of caregiver: health status (especially medical history and existence of chronic health conditions); other role responsibilities and perceived conflict with these roles; personal assessment of care burden; caregiving experience; ability to provide care; relationship with family members and other support systems; willingness to ask for and receive assistance; willingness to allow professional caregivers into the home; quality and history of relationship with care receiver; ability to deal with stress; spiritual resources; usual methods of coping including leisure patterns; presence of depression and grief	Provides baseline assessment; identifies problems or potential problems that require intervention

Interventions	Rationales	Interventions	Rationales
Assess home environment in the following areas: safety; access to medical equipment, professional caregivers, and emergency medical services; presence and appropriate use of adaptive equipment; cleanliness; availability of kitchen and bathroom facilities; appropriate space for care provision as well as continued family activities	Identifies problems that will require intervention; may identify need to find alternative care location (at the home of another relative or friend; long-term care facility; hospital, etc.)	Develop supportive and trusting relationship with caregiver: spend time discussing care problems with caregiver; provide empathetic interactions; promote a sense of competency; pay attention to caregiver needs; encourage caregiver to express negative emotions and provide support; reassess health and emotional status of caregiver and help caregiver to develop coping plans as needed	Necessary for support of caregiver, but may be met with resistance by caregiver who feels that "I'm not the patient. You're here to take care of my son/ daughter/spouse/ partner."
Assess for factors that contribute to caregiver role strain such as unrealistic expectations, poor insight, inability to use resources, unsatisfactory relationship with care receiver, insufficient resources (financial, respite, family, etc.), social isolation	Provides baseline; determines need for specific interventions	Teach caregiver to perform care activities in a safe, efficient, and energy conserving manner; provide demonstrations for all new activities and assist with interventions until caregiver feels secure	Decreases anxiety; promotes ability to rely on nursing support; increases feeling of competence in caregiving

Interventions	Rationales	Interventions	Rationales
Assist caregiver to identify needs related to home and yard care, shopping, meal preparation, finances, respite, medical treatments, ADLs for care receiver etc.; discuss resources that provide support (meals on wheels, homemaker services, in-home nursing care, social services, religious organizations, community HIV organizations, etc.); as determined by caregiver and care receiver, contact appropriate resources and initiate services	Maintains control and independence for caregiver while providing assistance with those services that s/he can relinquish; conserves energy resources so caregiver can focus on those activities deemed to have most importance	Enlist assistance of family and friends as is acceptable to caregiver and care receiver; help them understand the need for supportive interactions through letters, phone calls, and visits; support their efforts to provide care while allowing primary caregiver to spend time resting, relaxing, or pursuing leisure activities; encourage them to listen without offering advice; encourage them to offer assistance and then follow through on promises	Family is often an established source of trusted support; maintains family interactions; provides respite and emotional support for caregiver
		Encourage caregiver interaction in support groups for caregivers (frequently offered through community HIV organizations); assist with development of telephone or one-on-one interactions with caregivers who have experienced similar situations	Provides opportunity for mutual support and sharing of problems and solutions; demonstrates that caregiver does not have to do it all; supports ability to ask for assistance

Interventions	Rationales
Teach stress reduction strategies to caregiver and assist with development of a "time out" schedule; strategies may include, among others, exercise, relaxation tapes, visiting friends, shopping, attending religious services, reading, time management, meditation, or biofeedback	Encourages and provides permission for care of self
For HIV-infected caregivers, provide assistance in dealing with prospects of "watching what will eventually happen to me"; provide supportive care on a regular basis; encourage attention to personal health and stress levels; discuss issues related to anger, guilt, depression, fear, grief etc.; encourage continued participation in activities of personal interest; refer for medical and mental health care as needed	Acknowledges presence of personal health issues; encourages self-care; allows ventilation; provides respite

Evaluation:

The caregiver:

1. Provides safe, supportive care to the HIV-infected client
2. Acknowledges need for personal support and accesses resources in family and community
3. Shares frustrations about difficulty of care for significant other
4. Receives assistance from family members and/or professional caregivers

Ineffective Individual Coping

A state in which an individual experiences difficulties in meeting life's demands because of an impairment of adaptive and problem-solving abilities.

Related to:

Advancing HIV disease and associated physical and psychosocial disturbances; lifestyle changes required by increasing health problems; lack of a cure or clear treatment course; disruptions of relationships; poverty; inadequate support system; lack of resources; low self-esteem; perceived lack of control; stress overload; multiple losses; pain; hopelessness; powerlessness; culturally related conflicts with life experiences (especially sexual orientation, drug use, sex work, and HIV disease); loss of hope and/or spiritual values; social withdrawal

Defining Characteristics:

Ineffective coping

- **Subjective Findings:** Verbalizes inability to cope with situations related to advancing HIV infection; worries about inability to meet role expectations; reports overwhelming stress and anxiety; admits to an inability to ask for assistance and fear of becoming dependent; discusses increased use of drugs or alcohol as a coping mechanism; expresses hopelessness, sadness, pessimism, or lack of future orientation; states that current quality of life is unacceptable

- **Objective Findings:** Difficulty with problem solving and decision making; destructive behavior toward self or others; inability to meet basic needs; low self-esteem; impaired self-efficacy; inability to identify or access resources; low morale; lack of clear, realistic goals; hopelessness; social withdrawal; inflexible; hypervigilant; refuses assistance; does not maintain personal hygiene or ADLs; inappropriate behaviors in social situations

Outcome Criteria:

Enhanced ability to cope

Interventions/Rationales

Implement interventions discussed in Ineffective Individual Coping in Secondary Prevention.

Evaluation:

The client:

1. Discusses issues that cause coping problems
2. Acknowledges personal strengths and uses those strengths to plan coping strategies
3. Accepts support from nursing relationship and other resources
4. Develops coping plan and follows through with appropriate actions

Ineffective Denial

A state in which an individual consciously or unconsciously attempts to disavow progression of HIV disease in order to reduce anxiety or fear to the detriment of her/his health.

Related to:

Inability to acknowledge progression of HIV disease; prolonged treatment without cure; multiple losses; pre-existing or developing financial crisis related to expense of health care and/or loss of employment; alcohol or drug use; religious, social, or cultural sanctions related to sexuality, drug use, chronic disease, disability, and HIV infection

Defining Characteristics:

Inability to accept progression of HIV disease

- **Subjective Findings:** Denies that increasing symptoms are relevant, serious or dangerous; denies or cannot admit that advancing symptoms have an impact on capabilities and/or life pattern; dismisses importance of distressing symptoms or events; expresses feelings of inadequacy, guilt, loneliness, despair, fear, anxiety, stress, anger, frustration

- **Objective Findings:** Refuses to seek health care; distrusts health care system; unable or unwilling to list symptoms that need to be reported to health care providers in a timely manner; does not perceive dangers inherent in denial; uses unproven remedies to treat symptoms; minimizes symptoms; inappropriate affect

Outcome Criteria:

Acknowledges progression of HIV infection

Interventions	Rationales	Interventions	Rationales
Assess to determine diagnosis of Ineffective Denial: differentiate from nonadherence issues, lack of sufficient information, inability to understand information about HIV disease and its symptoms, avoidance (unwillingness to discuss or dwell on diagnosis or progressing symptoms); establish lack of fear related to advancing symptoms; determine that denial is ineffective over time (lack of direct actions for health care)	Provides important assessment information that may lead to focused interventions such as those described in Noncompliance (Nonadherence), Decisional Conflict, Anxiety, Fear, Hopelessness, Powerlessness, Self-Esteem Disturbance, Altered Family Processes, Grieving, Social Isolation, Altered Sexuality Patterns, Ineffective Individual Coping (above), and Spiritual Distress (below); also see Ineffective Denial in Secondary Prevention	Assess level of denial: high levels of denial are necessary for the client to control fear and anxiety; moderate or low levels of denial may indicate ability to express, discuss, and explore alternative coping mechanisms	Assists with intervention decisions
		Avoid direct confrontation of denial, especially at high levels; remain available and supportive	Reduces risk of entrenching denial; prevents destruction of therapeutic relationship; acknowledges the potential therapeutic effect of denial
Explore client's interpretation of the situation: what is happening to his/her health; what symptoms mean; which health care interventions are perceived to be appropriate, if any	Assesses knowledge base; provides input for planning future interventions; supports therapeutic relationship	Encourage client to discuss concerns, fears, and anxieties: provide a supportive, therapeutic, and safe relationship; never minimize client's expressed concerns; allow for sufficient time during which trust can be developed	Indirectly addresses the need for denial; provides opportunity for client to express concerns; allows continued relationship and opportunity for nursing interventions
		Correct client's inaccuracies and deficiencies in knowledge base; emphasize symptoms that need to be reported to health care providers in a timely manner	Clarifies information; supports reporting of problems; limits ability to use erroneous information as basis for denial

Interventions	Rationales
Address ethical issues that arise from client's denial in multidisciplinary groups that include medical ethicists and mental health professionals; develop united approach to client care based on group decisions; maintain client's right to self-determination as possible; include family or significant others in discussions as appropriate	Provides a forum for health care providers to express concerns and develop consensus on intervention efforts

Evaluation:

The client:

1. Maintains supportive relationship with nurse
2. Develops a knowledge base that supports reporting of symptoms
3. Experiences reduction in fear and/or anxiety

Ineffective Family Coping: Disabling

A state in which a family demonstrates destructive behaviors that disable the ability to adapt to the health challenge created by progressing HIV disease in one of the family members.

*Author's Note:

This diagnosis is useful in situations where (1) there is a pre-existing dysfunction in a family unit that then suffers the additional stress of HIV disease in a family member, or (2) the existence of advancing disease in a member of the family severely stresses the family's ability to cope and creates a dysfunctional state. This may be compounded in HIV disease where more than one member of the family may be infected. Other nursing diagnoses that may be more appropriate if family function has not become dysfunctional are Impaired Home Maintenance Management, Altered Family Processes, Parental Role Conflict, or Caregiver Role Strain which are discussed above and in previous sections. Remember that any intervention or coordination of care with family members must be done with the client's knowledge and consent. Some clients have already dealt with this issue and have developed alternative systems of support so that they will not have to deal with their families as their illness progresses. Other clients will feel the need at this point to re-establish relationships with family members. Remember that family is defined by the client and may or may not include blood- or marital-relatives. The nurse will need to assess the situation and provide interventions that support the client's needs and desires.

Related to:

Families with a history of dysfunction, abuse, substance use, emotional disturbance, or poor coping abilities; families that are unwilling or unable to meet psychosocial needs of their members; progressing HIV disease and related care needs; chronic, progressive, and debilitating course of HIV disease; decreasing ability of family member with HIV disease to care for self, contribute to family support, or maintain usual roles; unrealistic expectations of ability to provide support or continue responsibilities; anxiety; fear of stigma associated with HIV infection and social discrimination; lack of support from extended family, social networks, religious affiliations, etc.; ambivalent family relationships related to sexual orientation or drug use issues; multiple stressors and losses; refusal to access assistance from external resources; presence of an authoritarian family member; familial isolation; knowledge deficits

Defining Characteristics:

Ineffective family processes

- **Subjective Findings:** *Client* complains about neglect, abuse, indifference, rejection, intolerance, violence, or abandonment from family; develops helplessness and dependence; expresses concerns about family's ability to cope; *Family Member(s)* observe and report neglect, abuse, indifference, rejection, intolerance, violence, or abandonment toward client; report anxiety, depression, powerlessness, hopelessness, guilt, denial, anger, fear, blame, rejection, jealousy, agitation, hostility, aggression, inability to cope; over or underestimate capabilities of client and distort realities of the situation; take on symptoms of HIV

- **Objective Findings:** *Family Members* do not maintain contact as evidenced by a lack of visits, telephone calls, letters, etc.; inadequate care or support for HIV-infected client in home care situations; neglect; desertion; actions which are detrimental to client's physical, psychosocial, economic and/or health care status; demeaning remarks directed toward client; actions that promote dependence, low self-esteem, and helplessness in client; inadequate or unhealthy coping behaviors such as denial, abuse, increased substance use, etc.; lack of any signs of a meaningful or supportive family environment; inadequate knowledge and skills to provide care or support

Outcome Criteria:

Effective family coping; appropriate care and support for client with HIV infection

Interventions	Rationales
Develop supportive, trusting and therapeutic relationship with family members and significant others by spending time with each individual as possible; establish nursing role as one of facilitating assistance and support	Provides basis for all future assessment and intervention; encourages honest interactions
Perform continuing assessments of family: situation; composition; economics; culture; dynamics; coping behaviors; interaction patterns; connections to community; health beliefs; feelings related to HIV infection, sexual orientation, drug use; role assignment and performance; balance of power; health care needs; stressors; knowledge; resistance to assistance; etc.	Provides baseline for intervention development; allows early detection of changes and coping problems

Interventions	Rationales	Interventions	Rationales
Assess strengths and weaknesses related to coping with and/or caring for HIV-infected family member; verify perceptions with members of the family; encourage them to express feelings, concerns, problems, etc.; allow and support ventilation of anger, grief, pain; discourage blaming	Provides baseline data; provides insight into family dynamics and concerns; continues to establish rapport; establishes nurse as a person with whom discussion of problematic issues is safe	Help family appraise the situation: encourage family meetings to discuss issues (What problems have developed as a result of the advancing HIV disease of one family member? What new needs exist within the family and who will take on new responsibilities? What options exist? Can the family develop a plan that will meet the needs of all family members?); ask family members to develop empathy by asking them to imagine how they would feel if they were another family member; refer for family counseling as needed; as possible, include HIV-infected family member in all planning processes; encourage family members to share in necessary care and support duties	Establishes the family as the group that will evaluate problem and develop plans for coping; promotes group effort; decreases divisiveness; decreases individual burnout

Interventions	Rationales
Assess ability and willingness of the family to support and care for HIV-infected client	Establishes feasibility of family support and care; allows development of alternative plans for care and support if family is not able to participate
Teach family how to provide the needed care and support: instruct on home care requirements; provide demonstrations, practice time, and feedback for care tasks; reinforce emotionally caring behaviors and attitudes; discuss and provide reading materials about signs, symptoms, and treatments for HIV and opportunistic diseases; discuss and provide reading materials on pain management, nutrition, skin care, mouth care, etc.; supply lists of agencies that can provide resources such as respite care, support groups, counseling, nursing and homemaker services, financial support, etc.	Develops needed knowledge and skills; decreases stressors and fears related to care; promotes supportive interactions; identifies services that can be accessed for assistance

Interventions	Rationales
Provide supportive feedback: praise efforts and successes; point out increasing abilities and skills; correct techniques that are ineffective, inefficient, or dangerous; re-teach appropriate activities as needed; encourage client to express appreciation and praise as able	Increases feelings of self-efficacy, competence, and self-esteem; corrects problems in a supportive manner; encourages continued interactions

Evaluation:

The client:

1. Expresses satisfaction with family interactions
2. Expresses confidence and security in family abilities to provide support and/or care

The family:

1. Interacts in a supportive and caring manner
2. Demonstrates ability to provide care within limits specified by group consensus
3. Accesses and accepts available resources that promote ability to provide continued support and care to all family members

Relocation Stress Syndrome

A state in which the client suffers physical and/or psychosocial disturbance as a result of a transfer from one environment to another.

*Author's Note:

HIV symptom development signals the need for decisions about health care in a variety of environments. Care in a hospital intensive care unit or medical unit may be required for acute conditions that are short term in nature. Clients may also consider more permanent and substantial relocation efforts at this point: some will move to living centers designed for HIV-infected clients while others will move home to be closer to family and friends. Moving home may mean independent living quarters in the same community as family or may literally mean moving into the home of a relative. All of these moves create traumas related to acknowledgement of increasing disability and the losses inherent in such moves.

Related to:

Decreasing physical health and functioning; need for hospitalization or increased assistance in the home; decreased control of living arrangements; major differences between old and new environments; changes in levels of care; multiple losses experienced prior to and during relocation; abandonment requiring changes in environment in order to receive needed physical, social, and economic supports; lack of preparation and control of relocation

Defining Characteristics:

Acute stress related to relocation

- **Subjective Findings:** Verbalizes stress, discomfort, reluctance, insecurity, anger, anxiety, grief, and feelings of displacement; expresses feelings of increased dependency, loneliness, loss of identity, powerlessness, and uncertainty about the future; increases demands on family and caregivers; makes unfavorable comparisons between old and new environments

- **Objective Findings:** Changes in sleep and eating patterns; increasing dependence, questioning, and distrusting behaviors; restlessness; sad affect; aggressive behaviors; confusion and disorientation; withdrawal and detachment; withholds self from social interaction and attachment

Outcome Criteria:

Appropriate grief for losses and adjustment to new environment

Interventions	Rationales
Provide client with a supportive relationship that can be continued throughout change: arrange for follow-up visit(s) if possible; case management can follow client from facility to home and back; family or significant other may have to provide continuity during long-distance moves; develop trusting relationship with client as a prelude to preparation and education related to transfers	Establishes continuity during environment change; allows sharing of concerns and information

Interventions	Rationales
Identify areas of stress and loss related to relocation and assist client to deal with these issues as well as the relocation itself; initiate interventions discussed in Anxiety, Fear, Hopelessness, Powerlessness, Situational Low Self-Esteem, Grieving, Anticipatory Grieving, Social Isolation, and Ineffective Denial (above), as needed	Acknowledges that relocation is often accompanied by a wide variety of other issues; initiates interventions that may enhance client's ability to tolerate change
Initiate preparation for relocation as early as possible: discuss all changes with client; ask for and use client input; arrange for as much consistency in the environments as possible (i.e., maintain schedules, take personal affects, clothing, pictures, mementos, etc. to new location); introduce client to people in the new environment; with the client's consent, involve family members and significant others as much as possible	Provides opportunities for client control; maintains level of care; decreases anxiety about unknown

Interventions	Rationales
If moving in with family, friends, or others, provide support to new individuals in the client's environment; assess for concerns and potential problems; provide education about HIV disease and the client's care needs; teach infection control measures; identify community support systems	Supports individuals in the new environment; provides information to decrease anxiety and stressors related to accepting client into the living arrangements

Evaluation:

The client:

1. Acknowledges need for relocation
2. Takes an active part in planning for changes
3. Discusses concerns and grieves for losses
4. Becomes comfortable in new environment with a minimum of discomfort

Risk for Violence, Self-Directed

A state in which an individual is at risk of killing him/herself.

*Author's Note:

For some individuals with HIV infection, symptom development is the time when suicide becomes a viable option. Many who have dealt with the diagnosis and initial problems caused by the diagnosis are unable to cope when symptoms indicate advancing infection.

Related to:

Pervasively negative connotations in the general public related to HIV infection and AIDS; anger or grief related to poor response to ART; expectations of stigmatization and discrimination related to diagnosis and advancing disease; perceived inability to deal with disability and pain; lack of a cure; knowledge deficit related to course of HIV disease and treatment options; depression; ineffective coping skills; lack of support system

Defining Characteristics:

Death seen as the best solution

- **Subjective Findings:** Expresses desire to die; makes frequent statements such as "I should end it all before it gets any worse," "My family would be better off if I were dead," or "I can't live with the headaches/night sweats/fatigue"

- **Objective Findings:** History of suicidal ideation or suicide attempt, especially as a means to deal with life problems; depression; low self-esteem; hopelessness; helplessness; powerlessness; escalating substance use

Outcome Criteria:

Suicide attempt prevented

Interventions/Rationales

Initiate interventions discussed in Risk for Violence, Self-Directed in Secondary Prevention.

Evaluation:

The client:

1. Verbalizes intent to continue living

2. Accepts assistance from variety of resources

3. Develops effective alternative coping strategies

Spiritual Distress

A state of disruption in the individual's belief or value system that provides strength, hope, and meaning to life and that transcends the individual's biological and psychosocial nature.

Related to:

Advancing HIV disease; real or anticipated losses; pain; disability; social stigma; social isolation; terminal nature of HIV disease; multiple losses; feelings that spiritual system has failed; lack of previously developed spiritual values; denial of need for spirituality; separation from religious, cultural, or family ties; admission to a facility that prevents practice of spiritual rituals that require privacy, special diets, freedom from interruption, etc.

Defining Characteristics:

Searching for a spiritual base

- **Subjective Findings:** Questions belief system, relationship with higher power, personal significance, need for suffering; feels infection is incongruent with previously held beliefs; expresses ambivalence about beliefs; describes a sense of spiritual emptiness; initiates discussions about meaning of life, death, disease; relates history of negative response from religious leaders or congregations; expresses anger toward God; describes HIV as a punishment for previous behaviors; blames self or denies responsibility

- **Objective Findings:** Requests spiritual assistance, appetite and sleep disturbances, crying

Outcome Criteria:

Receives spiritual support and comfort

Interventions/Rationales

Initiate interventions described in Spiritual Distress in Secondary Prevention.

Evaluation:

The client:

1. Continues and/or enhances positive spiritual practices
2. Explores options for spiritual development and support
3. Expresses satisfaction with belief system and associated supports
4. Experiences enhanced inner peace and decreased somatic and emotional distress

Chapter VI

Terminal Care

The good news, as discussed in the Introduction, is that new drugs and treatment protocols have increased the quality and quantity of life for many HIV-infected people in developed countries all over the world. Recent successes have lead to optimism that HIV infection, if not curable, will at least be treatable for extended periods of time. In addition, new drugs and the possibility of improved therapeutic regimens are in development and will be released soon. The hope is that sometime in the near future there will no longer be a need for this chapter. Unfortunately, that is not the case at this time. There are still limits to the ability to treat HIV disease: some clients will not respond to drug therapy, some will not have access to the latest drugs or medical care, some will refuse to take the drugs, and some will suffer side effects (especially hepatic and renal complications) that will lead to death. And so, even though the need for terminal care issues related to HIV are decreasing in the United States, death and dying issues continue to be a concern for those involved in the care of HIV-infected clients.

Because HIV has a reputation for leading to death, infected clients—even in the early stages of disease—express concerns about the quality of care that will be available should they progress to a terminal state. They worry about becoming weak and losing the ability to care for themselves. In addition, family and friends will express concern about their abilities to provide increasingly intense supportive care for an HIV-infected loved one. Health care workers will focus on the increasing demands of a terminally ill client as well as on the personal stressors related to watching the death process in an individual who may have become important to the provider. All involved individuals, including the client, will experience frustration, anxiety, grief, and loss if the client's health status deteriorates.

These feelings escalate as death becomes imminent. Nursing care can become especially important during this time as the focus shifts to comfort and supportive care. The goals of nurse caring for HIV-infected clients in the terminal phase of illness are to:

1. Promote comfort: minimize disease symptoms, opportunistic disease, and side effects of treatment.
2. Allay loneliness and depression.
3. Maintain dignity.
4. Facilitate grief work.

These goals provide guidance for decision making in the terminal phase. New conditions will frequently emerge as the client's health deteriorates. The decision to aggressively treat these problems will be influenced not only by how effective the interventions may be, but also by the costs to the client and family. Costs must be measured in terms of economics, physical discomfort, and treatment requirements, which may require the client to move into an acute or chronic care facility in order to receive therapy. Often at this point in the disease process, clients and families do not want aggressive measures; on the other hand, some clients and families will want to have intensive therapy and interventions up to the very end. As possible, these decisions should be respected.

Nurse caring in the terminal phase of HIV disease can take place in any health care setting, including acute care facilities, long-term care facilities, and private homes. Hospice providers, working in all of these care locations as well as in hospice facilities, have supported many of these deaths. HIV-infected clients and their families have many choices for terminal care, but the growing trend is toward home care through the final phases of the disease with support as needed from health care professionals. In some communities, the majority of HIV-infected clients die at home. Home care through the terminal phases of any disease is dependent on the availability of support systems through families, friends, and professional nursing care agencies. Home care providers need assurances that health care institutions are willing to accept clients if emergencies arise or if changes occur that require institutionalized care for the client. These may include changes in attitude or ability to tolerate a death in the home, changes in the capabilities of care providers, changes in financial or insurance status that limits professional assistance in the home, or symptom changes that cannot be handled in the home setting.

Assessment

Nursing assessment is a continuing need during the terminal phase of care. Assessments should be related to the goals discussed above. Degree of comfort, for example, will direct many nursing interventions as will levels of loneliness, depression, and grief. A primary goal of many people in the terminal phase of life is to die with dignity. Nurses must continually assess whether this goal is being met or not. Frequent assessments of privacy issues, access to significant others (who may not be accepted by blood relatives), attention to wishes expressed in advanced directives (such as living wills and powers of attorney), and grooming and cleanliness concerns will allow nurses to re-direct care into more appropriate, client-centered interventions.

In addition, the nurse needs to monitor the client for symptoms of deterioration that may indicate impending death. Although the time of death can never be predicted, signs of deterioration should be shared with family members and significant others so that plans can be made. Often, out-of-town relatives and friends will not be notified until death appears to be close. If caregivers are

kept well informed, this may facilitate the process and provide them with needed support during the grief caused by the loss of the client.

Specific Nursing Diagnoses and Interventions

Ineffective Management of Therapeutic Regimen

A state in which the HIV-infected client experiences difficulty integrating treatments into his or her daily life.

*Author's Note:

The treatment of HIV infection in the final stages of life can require complex and confusing care that must now be facilitated by caregivers. Most often, the client will not be able to manage treatment regimens without the assistance of others.

Related to:

Complex therapeutic regimens; inability to understand requirements; lack of physical ability to carry out therapies; lack of assistance in the home; confusing health care system; costs of therapy; side effects of therapy; interactions of therapies; knowledge deficit; decisional conflicts; mistrust of therapies and/or health care providers

Defining Characteristics:

Inability to maintain therapeutic requirements

- **Subjective Findings:** States desire to maintain health care independently; discusses need for assistance that is not readily available; verbalizes feelings of being continually tired, causing an inability to complete personal care

- **Objective Findings:** Advancing symptoms that include fatigue, confusion, disorientation; frail and fragile appearance; lack of ability to maintain hygiene and cleanliness; doesn't return for appointments; lack of care support in the home; demonstrated inability to complete actions required in therapy; client may be bedfast, weak, incontinent, demented, or comatose

Outcome Criteria:

Has access to healthcare through support by significant others and/or professional health care providers

Interventions	Rationales
Initiate interventions described in Ineffective Management of Therapeutic Regimen in Tertiary Prevention	Provides assessment and initial intervention tactics

Interventions	Rationales
Teach client, significant others, and home care providers about each therapy: ascertain client and family expectations from the therapy; discuss potential benefits and side effects; provide written schedules and guidelines for medications and treatments; demonstrate equipment and require that client and/or family member provide return demonstrations for procedures; discuss follow-up/adjunct care required (i.e., regular lab monitoring); list complications that need to be reported immediately; assist with required modifications of home and lifestyle	Involves caregivers who will be providing increasing care; decreases knowledge deficit; provides information needed to make decisions and initiate therapy; establishes nurse as a knowledgeable and supportive resource
Prepare client and caregivers for changes in therapy as goals of care change: comfort, rest, and privacy issues may emerge as more important goals than medication regimens, for example; assist caregivers to assess situation and revise interventions	Promotes smooth transitions from earlier care issues to those important for terminal care

Interventions	Rationales
Support care providers: provide information and demonstrations for proper care; encourage "down time" and respite care; encourage verbalizations about frustrations of providing care, grief, and loss; focus on integrating care into the daily routines of the family	Establishes supportive resource for family, friends, and other care providers

Evaluation:

The client:

1. Receives needed care in a safe environment

Hyperthermia

A state in which the client's body temperature is elevated above her/his normal range.

Related to:

HIV infection; secondary infection(s); dehydration; medication reactions

Defining Characteristics:

Temperature greater than client's baseline (usually above 37.8° C/101° F orally or 38.8° C/102° F rectally)

- **Subjective Findings:** *Client or Significant Other* provides history of fever, recurrent night sweats, fatigue, vomiting, diarrhea, and/or symptoms of specific infectious processes such as coughing, headaches, sore throat, etc.

- **Objective Findings:** Elevated temperature; hot, flushed skin; diaphoresis; tachycardia; tachypnea; altered mental status including decreased levels of alertness, cognition, and orientation; dehydration manifested by dry skin, poor skin turgor, decreased fluid intake and output, concentrated urine

Outcome Criteria:

Temperature maintained within baseline norms

Interventions/Rationales

Initiate interventions described in Hyperthermia in Tertiary Prevention; focus at this point may be less on diagnosis of causes of increased temperature and more on comfort and safety measures.

Evaluation:

The client:

1. Maintains body temperature within normal range
2. Remains comfortable and safe during fever episode

Fluid Volume Deficit

A state in which the client experiences vascular, cellular, or intracellular dehydration.

Related to:

Nausea; vomiting; malabsorption related to HIV enteropathy; diarrhea; fever; increased metabolic rate; systemic infection(s); decreased motivation to drink fluids related to painful lesions in the mouth, depression, apathy, fatigue; anorexia; difficulty swallowing; diaphoresis

Defining Characteristics:

Negative balance of intake and output; insufficient oral intake

- **Subjective Findings:** *Client or Significant Other* reports excessive vomiting, diarrhea, fever, night sweats, decreased urine output; *Client* complains of thirst, dry mouth, dry skin, dizziness or lightheadedness, difficulty in swallowing, and/or painful lesions in mouth

- **Objective Findings:** Weight loss; signs of dehydration: poor skin turgor, pallor, orthostatic hypotension, elevated temperature, tachycardia; dry skin and mucous membranes; concentrated urine; client may be comatose or semi-comatose and unable to swallow fluids

Outcome Criteria:

Adequate hydration

Interventions	Rationales
Initiate interventions described in Fluid Volume Deficit in Tertiary Prevention; at this point, focus is on comfort and less on diagnostic procedures	Provides assessment and interventions that help to alleviate problems related to dehydration
If acceptable to the client and family, administer IV fluids and electrolytes as ordered: maintain patent IV access, monitor flow rates (rapid replacement may be required), monitor client response	Provides replacement of fluids and electrolytes

Evaluation:

The client:

1. Replaces fluid losses
2. Remains comfortable despite fluid balance problems

Fluid Volume Excess

A state in which the client experiences increased fluid retention and edema.

Related to:

Side effects of medications; immobility; poor intake of protein; excess intake of sodium; inadequate lymphatic drainage due to lymphatic occlusion caused by HIV, KS, other cancers and infections; liver disease related to past history of hepatitis, cirrhosis, malignancy, or side effect to ART

Defining Characteristics:

Edema, especially in dependent areas

- **Subjective Findings:** *Client or Significant Other* points out areas of taut, shiny skin over areas of swelling; *Client* complains of pain in regions of edema

- **Objective Findings:** Areas of edema, especially in dependent areas (legs and feet in clients who are ambulatory; legs, feet, and sacral areas for clients who spend a large part of the day sitting up; sacral areas in bedfast clients); weight gain; shortness of breath may indicate progression to congestive heart failure; decreasing urine output

Outcome Criteria:

Comfort and intact skin

Interventions	Rationales	Interventions	Rationales
Assess for edema by observing areas of potential edema on a daily basis: note presence of swelling and condition of skin; weigh daily; listen to lung fields on a daily basis (and more often as needed) to detect congestion	Provides baseline assessment as well as early indication of developing problems	Prevent dependent venous pooling: maintain mobility as long as possible; turn often if on bed rest; elevate extremities above the level of the heart in an extended position; provide complete support for elevated extremities with pillows under entire length; elevate head of bed if face is edematous; avoid bed rest positions that maintain sacral area in lowest position; avoid constrictive articles of clothing, especially socks and stockings; consider use of support hose	Improves lymph drainage; decreases cardiac work to return fluids to the heart; enhances renal perfusion and elimination
Report problems to care provider; assist with development of medical care plan; provide appropriate interventions; monitor electrolyte components in IV fluids; monitor protein available through oral, tube, or IV feedings; monitor output; administer diuretics or albumin, as ordered, and observe for effects on client; monitor electrolytes and ABGs	Provides input for medical interventions that may decrease risk of edema and/or reverse existing edema; aggressive treatment of edema may not be tolerated by the client at this point: client and family desires should be considered when making plans for any new therapy during the terminal phase	Protect skin: see Impaired Skin Integrity in Tertiary Prevention	Prevents skin breakdown and pain associated with skin problems
		Monitor dietary intake and encourage appropriate changes: increase intake of proteins, decrease intake of foods high in sodium; balance these requirements with client food preferences and ability to maintain necessary nutritional intake; encourage 6 small meals per day	Maintains nutritional intake while adjusting nutrients to prevent or decrease edema

Evaluation:

The client:

1. Exhibits a decrease in edema
2. Maintains skin integrity
3. Remains comfortable

Risk for Infection Transmission

A state in which the HIV-infected client is at risk for transmitting HIV to others. The focus during the terminal phase is on preventing HIV transmission to care providers.

Related to:

Lack of knowledge; accidents in which others come into contact with client's blood; denial; sharing of injection equipment; unprotected sexual intercourse

Defining Characteristics:

Continued risk to others

- **Subjective Findings:** Sexual and drug using activities usually decrease at this point in the client's life, but reports of unprotected sexual activity or sharing equipment when injecting drugs need to be addressed

- **Objective Findings:** Diagnosis of HIV infection; refuses to disclose HIV status to caregivers; increased need for care provision that may involve the risk of contact with blood or bloody fluids

Outcome Criteria:

Safe provision of appropriate care

Interventions/Rationales

Initiate interventions described in Risk for Infection Transmission in Secondary Prevention; focus should be on the use of UPs or BSI by all health care providers.

Evaluation:

The client:

1. Continues to receive appropriate care

Caregivers:

1. Discuss fears related to becoming infected while providing care
2. Demonstrate care using appropriate protective measures
3. Have access to appropriate equipment and instruction
4. Provide care in a safe and effective manner

Altered Nutrition: Less than Body Requirements

A state in which the client experiences weight loss related to inadequate intake and/or increased metabolism of nutrients.

*Author's Note:

Wasting and malnutrition frequently accompany the terminal phases of life. At this point, however, nutritional intake may not be the highest priority for the client and her or his significant others. The nurse will need to assess the situation and provide supportive nutritional care as tolerated by the client.

Related to:

Increased need for nutrient intake due to chronic infectious and/or neoplastic disease process(es); hypermetabolic state caused by infection(s), decreased ability to take food in related to mouth and esophageal lesions, nausea, vomiting, anorexia, apathy, depression, dementia, or coma; decreased ability to absorb nutrients in the GI tract; diarrhea; GI tract infections or cancers; decreased ability to obtain, prepare, or safely store food because of problems related to transportation, economics, fatigue, lack of social support, impaired cognition, immobility; knowledge deficit; side effects of medications

Defining Characteristics:

Loss of 10% or more of ideal body mass

- **Subjective Findings:** Complains of lack of appetite, altered taste sensations, discomfort when eating related to mouth sores, difficulty swallowing, nausea, vomiting, diarrhea and/or abdominal cramping; reports weight loss; describes economic or psychosocial problems that decrease ability to purchase and prepare food

- **Objective Findings:** Weight loss; wasted appearance; mental confusion; oral exam reveals mouth lesions and/or advanced gingivitis; lesions in throat; abnormal bowel sounds; inability to feed self; skin, hair, and nail changes that indicate malnutrition; triceps skin fold, mid-arm circumference, and mid-arm muscle circumference less than 60% of standard; muscle weakness and tenderness; knowledge deficit related to nutrition; lab work reveals decreased serum albumin levels and a negative nitrogen balance

Outcome Criteria:

Adequate nutritional intake

Interventions/Rationales

Initiate interventions discussed in Altered Nutrition: Less than Body Requirements in Tertiary Prevention; anticipate increased need for nutritional supplementation through feeding tubes and/or IV fluids; focus may now shift to maintaining fluid intake in order to promote comfort.

Evaluation:

The client:

1. Maintains adequate nutritional intake for metabolic needs
2. Remains comfortable

Impaired Swallowing

A state in which the client has decreased ability to voluntarily pass fluids and/or solid foods from the mouth to the stomach.

Related to:

Infectious and/or neoplastic lesions of the mouth, throat, esophagus; fatigue; depression; dementia and decreasing nervous system capabilities; coma

Defining Characteristics:

Difficulty or pain on swallowing

- **Subjective Findings:** *Client* describes feeling of fullness and pain behind the sternum; refuses to eat because of pain; expresses fear at the possibility of aspiration or choking; *Client* or *Caregiver* reports coughing, choking, or other problems when swallowing

- **Objective Findings:** Decreased intake; grimaces when swallowing; weight loss; holds food or fluids in oral cavity; signs of inadequate nutritional intake; signs of decreasing mental state or coma

Outcome Criteria:

Decreased pain and improved ability to swallow

Interventions/Rationales

Initiate interventions described in Impaired Swallowing in Tertiary Prevention; focus should now be on comfort and safety measures; anticipate increased use of IV fluids to maintain hydration.

Evaluation:

The client:

1. Remains comfortable
2. Receives necessary medications and fluids through alternative sources if swallowing is not possible or creates a risk of aspiration

Altered Oral Mucous Membranes

A state in which the client experiences change or disruption to the oral mucous membranes.

Related to:

Opportunistic diseases including candidiasis, herpes simplex, oral hairy leukoplakia, KS; primary HIV infection; poor oral hygiene; overgrowth of normal flora; malnutrition; dehydration; reactions to drug or local radiation therapy; periodontal disease; continued use of alcohol and tobacco; mouth breathing related to nasal and sinus infections; knowledge and/or skill deficits to perform appropriate mouth care

Defining Characteristics:

Disrupted oral mucous membranes

- **Subjective Findings:** Complains of dryness, bleeding, soreness, or burning in mouth or throat; reports changes in taste, pain when eating, or difficulty swallowing; reveals variety of lesions or inflamed areas in oral cavity; verbalizes difficulty in eating spicy or salty foods

- **Objective Findings:** Variety of lesions in oral cavity: white patchy areas, red-purple raised lesions, bleeding and inflamed gums, loose or missing teeth; halitosis; dry, cracked lips; diagnostic tests can provide identification of source of a number of pathogens or KS; enlarged lymph nodes in the neck

Outcome Criteria:

Intact oral mucous membranes that are free from irritation and pain

Interventions/Rationales

Initiate interventions described in Altered Oral Mucous Membranes in Tertiary Care; focus may now move to providing mouth care for the weakening client.

Evaluation:

The client:

1. Receives thorough oral care on a routine basis
2. Experiences maximum oral comfort
3. Maintains intact mucous membranes

Altered Bowel Elimination: Diarrhea

A state in which the client experiences a change in normal bowel habits, characterized by the frequent passage of loose, fluid, unformed stools.

Related to:

Gastrointestinal infections caused by HIV, *Giardia lamblia, Salmonella, Shigella, Campylobacter, Isospora belli, Cryptosporidium,* MAC, CMV, herpes simplex, or any other common GI tract pathogen; KS lesions in the GI tract; lactose intolerance; nutritional problems; intolerance to dietary supplements with a high osmolarity (either by mouth or NG tube); gastritis; irritable bowel; side effect to drug or radiation therapy

Defining Characteristics:

Frequent expulsion of loose or liquid stool

- **Subjective Findings:** Complains of passing loose stools frequently during the day, abdominal pain, cramping, or urgency; reports weakness, lack of appetite, and signs of dehydration; discusses fears of becoming incontinent and having to depend on others for care

- **Objective Findings:** Signs of dehydration; electrolyte imbalances; tenderness on abdominal palpation; hyperactive bowel sounds; documentation of stool losses of up to 12 liters of fluid per day; perianal excoriation; stool examination may provide diagnosis of pathogens

Outcome Criteria:

Control of diarrhea and complications of diarrhea

Interventions/Rationales

Initiate interventions described in Altered Bowel Elimination: Diarrhea in Tertiary Care; focus now is on maintaining cleanliness, preventing skin breakdown, and maintaining fluid and nutritional status.

Evaluation:

The client:

1. Experiences reduced frequency of stools
2. Maintains intact skin and mucous membranes in perianal region
3. Maintains adequate hydration, nutrition, and comfort levels

Urinary Elimination: Functional Incontinence

A state in which the client experiences involuntary, unpredictable passage of urine.

Related to:

Environmental problems that make it difficult to reach bathroom; change in environment; use of side rails; impaired mobility; fecal impaction; sensory deficits; cognitive deficits; disorientation, confusion, depression, progressive dementia; weakness; urinary tract infection; inability to communicate needs; inattentive caregivers; lack of available assistance

Defining Characteristics:

Urinary incontinence

- **Subjective Findings:** *Client* or *Caregiver* reports multiple episodes of urinary incontinence; *Client* verbalizes feelings of embarrassment, shame, or guilt at inability to maintain usual toileting practices and continence

- **Objective Findings:** Changes in health status that decrease ability to maintain usual toileting practices, including weakness, confusion, disorientation, change in environment; lack of appropriate or accessible bathroom facilities; repeated episodes of urinary incontinence; need for bedrest

Outcome Criteria:

Control of incontinence episodes

Interventions	Rationales
Assess incontinence problems: encourage client, caregiver, and/or family members to maintain records of incontinence episodes for 2-4 days; observe timing, frequency, amount of urine, and precursors to incontinent events; monitor intake and output records; assess for signs of urinary tract infection or fecal impaction	Provides baseline for intervention; identifies incontinence pattern; identifies treatable problems

Interventions	Rationales
Evaluate environment for bathroom access problems: How distant is the bathroom? Are there obstructions in the path to the bathroom? Are bed rails in the way? Does the bathroom have safety features such as no-skid rugs, hand bars, and good lighting? Are alternatives to the bathroom provided (i.e., bedside commodes, urinals, and bedpans)?	Provides information to develop interventions
Evaluate client ability to maintain toileting, look for the following problems: weakness; decreasing mobility and/or upper body strength; confusion; disorientation; vision problems; loss of balance; decreasing levels of consciousness	Provides information to develop interventions

Interventions	Rationales	Interventions	Rationales
Remove or reduce environmental problems: provide uncluttered access to bathroom; install safety features in the bathroom; provide with bedside commode, urinal, or bedpan as needed; keep bed in low position with siderails down if not required for safety; be readily available to assist with ambulation to the bathroom or transfer to a bedside commode; provide with easy-to-remove clothing for more rapid access to elimination receptacle	Increases access to proper receptacles for urinary elimination	Initiate use of external catheter for male clients	Provides noninvasive measure to maintain control of urine
		Place incontinence pads on bed as needed	Assists with the maintenance of a clean and dry bed surface
		Remove fecal impactions as needed; initiate bowel management program	Pressure of an impaction may be contributing to the problems with urinary incontinence
Initiate interventions described in Activity Intolerance and Fatigue in Tertiary Prevention	Maintains mobility; decreases problems related to progressive weakness	Maintain integrity of the skin: clean and dry perineal area well after each incontinent episode; observe area for signs of irritation and early breakdown; implement appropriate nursing care for problems; collaborate with primary care providers as needed	Prevents skin breakdown; decreases risk of opportunistic skin/ genital infections
Provide elimination reminders every 2 hours during the day, after meals, and before bedtime	Reminds clients with confusion or disorientation about need to void		
Provide with incontinence pads or pants	Decreases anxiety and embarrassment at incontinence episodes		

Interventions	Rationales
Support family caregivers in their efforts to maintain client dignity and cleanliness: discuss the importance of providing support to the client in this area; allow them to vent frustration and feelings of embar-rassment; listen and provide suggestions to decrease difficul-ties expressed; pro-vide respite care; arrange for profes-sional assistance in the home setting	Incontinence is a primary reason for admission to long-term care facilities; supporting family caregivers may allow the client to remain at home for terminal care; elimination and exposure of genital areas may be highly stressful to family members or friends who are providing care

Evaluation:

The client:

1. Maintains urinary continence or decreases numbers of incontinent episodes
2. Maintains integrity of skin and mucous membranes
3. Receives assistance for toileting and cleanliness

Disuse Syndrome

A state in which the client is at risk for deterioration of body systems as a result of prescribed or unavoidable musculoskeletal inactivity.

*Author's Note:

Inactivity can affect all body systems and organs. Thorough systems assessment is, therefore, more important at this point. All of the problems caused by Disuse Syndrome can be alleviated by increased activity. Related nursing diagnoses include Risk for Infection, Impaired Skin Integrity, Activity Intolerance, Altered Respiratory Function, Sensory Perceptual Alteration, Powerless-ness, and Body Image Disturbance—all of which are covered in Tertiary Prevention. Please refer to these specific diagnoses as needed. This diagnosis also includes the nursing diagnoses of Risk for Injury, Impaired Physical Mobility, Altered Tissue Perfusion, and Constipation.

Related to:

Decreasing levels of consciousness including coma; end-stage disease; major depression; medical equipment such as urinary catheters and intravenous lines; fatigue, debilitation, pain; medications

Defining Characteristics:

Presence of factors that contribute to immobility

- **Subjective Findings:** Complains of inabil-ity to "get around"; verbalizes frustrations related to decreasing activity, social inter-actions, intellectual stimulation; note: clients in terminal phases of disease may need this gradual withdrawal from inter-action and activity

- **Objective Findings:** Increasing depen-dence on caregivers for motion; orthostatic hypotension; weakness; confusion; muscle atrophy; evidence of decreasing brain and skin perfusion; areas of redness or break-down over bony prominences; abnormal joint positions that may lead to contrac-tures; dependent edema; developing complications such as emboli, compro-mised respiratory status, urinary retention, constipation, cardiovascular deterioration

Outcome Criteria:

Improved mobility and prevention of complications

Interventions	Rationales
Assess body systems while routinely focusing on problems related to immobility, especially skin, respirations, cardiovascular function, range of motion, elimination	Provides baseline and early detection of problems; establishes recognition of need for intervention
Maintain mobility at highest possible levels: encourage ambulation at regular intervals throughout the day; provide for chair rest as an alternative to staying in bed all day; encourage active range of motion exercises; provide passive range of motion exercise as needed; assist to reposition every 1-2 hours; consult with physical therapy	Mobility provides positive influences for all body systems; decreases risk of complication development (this intervention is understood to be an important component of all of the following interventions)

Interventions	Rationales
Maintain optimal respiratory function: encourage deep breathing and controlled coughing exercises with or without spirometry for 5 minutes every hour; auscultate lung fields on a routine basis; position with head up	Facilitates lung expansion; decreases risk of complications; allows early recognition of developing problems
Maintain integrity of skin: observe for reddened areas; position client with weight off of these areas as much as possible; maintain adequate nutrition and fluid intake; keep skin clean and dry; support extremities and back with cushions and pillows while in bed	Allows early recognition of problems; increases circulation to affected areas; prevents further deterioration
Enhance circulatory function: elevate extremities	Decreases blood pooling

Interventions	Rationales
Maintain bowel function: encourage adequate food and fluid intake; establish regular times for elimination, if 2 days go by without bowel movement, consult with primary care provider to obtain order for laxatives or enemas; provide for privacy; encourage use of bathroom or bedside commode; if bedpan is required, position in as much of an upright position as possible; check for and remove impactions as needed	Encourages usual bowel elimination
Include client and family as much as possible in planning and intervention: explain need for maintaining mobility; demonstrate interventions and ask for return demonstrations, including active and passive range of motion exercises, deep breathing, turning, and positioning	Involves all participants and encourages their cooperation; involves family and significant others in care process

Interventions	Rationales
Provide emotional support to client and family as mobility levels decrease: encourage expressions of anger, fear, fatigue, frustration, and grief; discuss issues as they arise; maintain hope but provide honest assessments of the client's condition; provide for respite care	Acknowledges difficulties associated with mobility-related losses; provides support as deterioration progresses

Evaluation:

The client:

1. Maintains body function status as long as possible
2. Receives care to prevent complications of disuse
3. Receives emotional support from all caregivers as condition deteriorates

The family/significant other:

1. Remains invested in client care
2. Receives emotional and physical support to continue care

Impaired Home Maintenance Management

A state in which the individual and/or family is unable to independently maintain a safe, care-providing environment for the HIV-infected client.

*Author's Note:

Home health care is becoming the norm for terminal care of HIV-infected clients in many communities. Supportive home health care requires assistance from a variety of family and community resources. An accepting and supportive family, while not absolutely necessary for home care, is an important component of successful terminal home care.

Related to:

Activity intolerance; chronic, debilitating disease; disuse syndrome; financial problems; lack of information about local resources; self-care deficit; inadequate support system; impaired mental status; substance use; inadequate housing or furnishings; inadequate community services; anticipatory grief; ineffective grieving

Defining Characteristics:

Inadequate home environment for appropriate care during terminal phase of HIV disease

- **Subjective Findings:** *Client* expresses concerns and/or fear related to staying at home during terminal disease; discusses financial difficulties related to housing; reports lack of assistance at home; complains of fatigue or weakness; demonstrates inadequate knowledge or skills to administer medications and prescribed treatments; *Client* or *Family* verbalizes difficulty in maintaining housekeeping, a safe environment, home repair

- **Objective Findings:** Observations that indicate problems with maintaining a safe, clean environment; demonstrated inability to care for self in home and/or to complete ADLs (including the maintenance of adequate nutrition); lack of connection with local resources and support systems;

lack of adequate safety devices such as ramps and handrails; lack of adequate heating, cooling, lighting, kitchen, or bathroom facilities; absence of transportation; dirty environment and/or the presence of insects or rodents; dangerous neighborhood

Outcome Criteria:

Improved home environment that promotes a comfortable and familiar environment during the terminal process

Interventions/Rationales

Implement interventions described in Impaired Home Maintenance Management in Tertiary Prevention; focus is on supporting family members and caregivers, assuring comfort and dignity for the client, and assisting with feelings related to loss and grief.

Evaluation:

The client or family/significant other:

1. Demonstrates ability to access supports needed to continue care in the home
2. Demonstrates skills required to continue care in the home
3. Requests and receives necessary assistance
4. Expresses satisfaction with housing, support services, and home situation

Self-Care Deficit Syndrome

A state in which the client experiences an impaired motor or cognitive function that causes a decreased ability to perform or complete activities of daily living in the following areas: feeding, bathing/hygiene, dressing/grooming, and toileting.

Related to:

Activity intolerance, fatigue, weakness, decreased strength and endurance; pain; presence of medical equipment such as urinary catheters, intravenous lines, feeding tubes, and/or oxygen masks; impaired vision; depression; grief; loss of motivation; severe anxiety; immobility; cognitive impairment; decreasing cognitive abilities; dementia; coma

Defining Characteristics:

Loss of or decreasing abilities to perform self-care activities

- **Subjective Findings:** *Client* or *Family* discusses decreasing abilities to maintain personal levels of hygiene, nutrition, toileting, and grooming

- **Objective Findings:** *Feeding:* demonstrates impaired ability to prepare food or introduce food into the mouth; *Bathing:* demonstrates an inability or unwillingness to wash body, comb hair, brush teeth, clean nails, etc.; *Dressing:* demonstrates inability to put on or take off usual daytime clothes, demonstrates difficulty in managing buttons, snaps, or other clothing closures; *Toileting:* demonstrates inability to get to a toilet in time for bladder or bowel evacuation, demonstrates inability to properly cleanse perineal area after elimination

Outcome Criteria:

Carries out ADLs independently or with assistance

Interventions	Rationales
Assess limitations of self-care abilities; determine causes of limitations, if possible	Provides baseline data and information for interventions; reassessment provides evaluation of improving or decreasing abilities
Promote client/family involvement in care as follows: share assessment findings with client and discuss compensation measures as the care plan is developed; provide choices as to time and method for daily care; encourage and allow client to provide as much self-care as possible, making adjustments for time as needed; provide updates on assessments and engage client in approving variations of care plan; as approved by the client, involve family and friends in discussions and provision of care	Supports self-esteem and feelings of control; encourages cooperation in the care process; allows continuation of self-care as possible

Interventions	Rationales	Interventions	Rationales
Enhance self-esteem and dignity: provide for privacy during toileting, bathing, and dressing procedures; provide assistance with actions and attitudes that communicate respect of the client and her or his body; allow client to direct the situation as much as possible	Reminds client and family caregivers of the dignity of life in difficult and/or embarrassing situations	Assist client to eat: determine client food likes and dislikes; provide for pain and/or nausea relief prior to meals; position client in a comfortable, upright position for eating; encourage family and friends to create a pleasant atmosphere for shared meals; place food and utensils in a convenient manner; cut foods into bite-size pieces and open packaged foods if client cannot do this; if full assistance is needed, allow client to direct the order in which foods are presented; plan on increased time for eating and allow sufficient time for chewing and swallowing, provide straws and other assistive eating devices as needed; also see Altered Nutrition: Less than Body Requirements and Fluid Volume Deficit (above)	Supports nutritional intake; decreases risk of malnutrition; supports personal control
Provide treatments that help to alleviate problems with care (i.e., medications for pain or anxiety; utilization of assistive devices for ambulation, hearing, and vision; orientation cues; catheter care; etc.)	Decreases underlying problems; enhances ability to continue involvement in self-care		

Interventions	Rationales	Interventions	Rationales
Assist client in bathing/hygiene measures: assess need for assistance and safety measures; determine client's preferred time, sequence, and methods for bathing and hygiene, conform to these preferences as possible; assure safety in the bathtub or shower with handrails, shower chairs, slip-protection mats, and observation as needed; place hygiene utensils (soap, towels, shampoo, razor, tooth brush, deodorant, etc.) in an easy-to-reach position; assist with hard-to-reach areas and/or fatiguing procedures, especially perineal cleaning and tooth brushing and flossing, as needed	Provides appropriate hygiene measures while supporting client control; provides assistance as needed while encouraging continued self-care; prevents injury; prevents infection problems related to poor hygiene; promotes good oral hygiene	Provide assistance with dressing/ grooming: determine client's clothing preferences and place selected clothing in an accessible location; encourage the use of clothing that is comfortable; encourage the use of clothing that is easy to remove for toileting purposes; encourage clothing that is as close to usual daytime wear as possible; provide for privacy while dressing, but be available to assist with difficult movements; place grooming equipment (hair brushes, razors, make up, etc.) in a convenient, easy-to-reach place; teach grooming and bathing methods that conserve energy and compensate for client limitations	Assures that the client is clothed and groomed in the manner to which she or he would normally conform; enhances self-esteem and body image; reinforces control and individuality

Interventions	Rationales
Assist with toileting activities: respond immediately to requests for assistance to prevent accidents; provide for privacy; provide care in a nonjudgmental manner, especially after incontinent episodes; provide toileting reminders at regular intervals to prevent accidents; maintain use of bathroom facilities as long as possible; assist client to adjust to assistive devices such as bedside commodes, bedpans, and/or urinals as needed; assist with clothing removal and readjustment before and after toileting; provide with appropriate materials for cleansing of perineal area after elimination, assist with this care as needed; discuss use of external catheters with male clients as needed	Maintains dignity as much as possible; prevents or decreases number of incontinent episodes; provides hygiene and comfort; prevents problems with elimination

Interventions	Rationales
If client is unable to provide self-care: engage family and friends to assist with ADLs; demonstrate methods of care and get return demonstrations; provide continuing assistance with care until caregivers express comfort with new tasks; assist caregivers to find professional support through home care providers; provide emotional support to caregivers as client's condition changes	Enhances relationships with family caregivers; provides needed care to the client; promotes self-efficacy among caregivers while maintaining supportive measures; assures caregivers that they are an important and needed part of the client's life

Evaluation:

The client:

1. Maintains control of self-care processes as long as possible
2. Receives all needed care despite decreasing abilities
3. Is assisted to maintain appropriate levels of nutrition, cleanliness, grooming, and elimination
4. Maintains self-respect and dignity

The family/significant other:

1. Perceives the importance of personal care and client control issues
2. Assists with care in an appropriate manner and to the best of their capabilities
3. Receives the support needed to provide care as client abilities decrease

Instrumental Self-Care Deficit

A state in which the client experiences a decreased ability to perform activities or access services needed to maintain a household.

Related to:

Terminal illness and advancing disease; muscular weakness; lack of coordination; visual disorders; depression; fatigue; decreasing strength and endurance; immobility; neurocognitive deficits including dementia; use of medical devices including equipment for intravenous fluids and medications, feeding tubes, long-term venous access devices; inadequate support systems

Defining Characteristics:

Inability to maintain independence in home setting without assistance

- **Subjective Findings:** Verbalizes fears about maintaining self at home, especially related to food preparation, shopping, house cleaning, laundry, money management, safety, transportation, and medication administration

- **Objective Findings:** Weakness; confusion; lack of social and economic supports; lack of hygienic living conditions; lack of appropriate kitchen facilities; nonadherence to medication regimen; missed clinic appointments

Outcome Criteria:

Safe and effective management of at-home care

Interventions/Rationales

Initiate interventions described in Instrumental Self-Care Deficit in Tertiary Prevention; focus now should be on supporting family and home care providers with education, emotional support, respite care, physical assistance, grief issues, financial matters, etc.

Evaluation:

The client:

1. Remains in home with appropriate support
2. Maintains as much independence as possible
3. Receives appropriate care in a safe manner

The family, friends, and home caregivers:

1. Provide appropriate supportive care and assistance
2. Receive necessary emotional, physical, social, and financial support

Sleep Pattern Disturbance

A state in which disturbances in the quantity or quality of rest patterns causes discomfort or interferes with the client's desired lifestyle.

*Author's Note:

The need for rest and increased sleep time are usual responses in the terminal phases of any disease process. The client's family may need assistance in supporting the client's need for more rest time because it may signify advancing disease to them. These periods of sleep may allow the client's significant others time to work on grief and loss issues.

Related to:

Anxiety; pain; diarrhea; night sweats; chills; treatment schedules; respiratory or circulatory disorders; bladder infections with associated frequency or incontinence; immobility; medications (especially sedatives, hypnotics, antidepressants, tranquilizers, amphetamines, corticosteriods, decongestants, caffeine, alcohol); lack of exercise or change in activity pattern; lifestyle disruptions (related to end of life issues); environmental changes such as living conditions, living companions, moving to a new environment, etc.; stress; depression; grief

Defining Characteristics:

Difficulty falling or remaining asleep

- **Subjective Findings:** Complains of difficulty in falling asleep, staying asleep, fatigue on awakening, not feeling rested, general fatigue; discusses problems with energy levels and staying awake during the day

- **Objective Findings:** Agitation, mood alterations; increasing irritability; decreased attention span; disorientation; lethargy; listlessness; decreased social interaction; frequent yawning; drooping eyelids and posture

Outcome Criteria:

Adequate rest

Interventions/Rationales

Initiate interventions described in Sleep Pattern Disturbance in Tertiary Prevention.

Evaluation:

The client:

1. Describes activities that can enhance sleep and rest
2. Obtains adequate rest to balance energy needs
3. Expresses satisfaction with sleep patterns

Pain

A state in which the client experiences the presence of severe discomfort and/or uncomfortable sensations.

Related to:

Opportunistic infections and malignancies; lymphadenopathy; edema and pressure; skin, oral, and/or genital lesions; side effects of therapies, especially radiation and drug-related peripheral neuropathy; arthralgia; myalgia; vasculitis; inflammation; chronic demyelinating neuropathy

Defining Characteristics:

Subjective experience of pain

- **Subjective Findings:** Verbal expressions of pain: pain is what, where, and how often the client says it is; complains of headaches, muscle aches, stiff neck, cramping abdominal pain, irritation around mucous membrane lesions

- **Objective Findings:** Protective or guarding behaviors such as splinting and posture; self-focused; altered perceptions of time and space; social withdrawal; impaired thought processes; moaning, crying, whimpering, pacing, restlessness, irritability; facial features including grimacing, clenched teeth, clenched jaw, knotted brow; muscle tension; changes in blood pressure, pulse, respirations; diaphoresis; dilated pupils

Outcome Criteria:

Pain relieved, controlled, or eliminated

Interventions/Rationales

Initiate interventions described in Pain in Tertiary Prevention.

Evaluation:

The client:

1. Identifies precipitating or aggravating factors to pain and develops coping mechanisms to moderate these experiences
2. Uses preferred pharmacologic and non-pharmacologic mechanisms to assist with pain relief
3. Discusses episodes of pain with the nurse
4. Verbalizes a decrease in the intensity and duration of pain episodes

Decisional Conflict

A state of indecision between competing choices that involve risk, loss, or challenge to established personal lifestyle or values.

Related to:

Dementia; social withdrawal; physical discomforts; indecision related to end-of-life issues; confusing, inconsistent, or incomplete information related to treatment options, legal, and social issues; disagreement within support system about best course(s) to take as chances of survival decrease; inexperience in decision making; unclear personal value system or a conflict with personal values; ethical dilemmas related to sexuality or drug use; resignation; hopelessness

Defining Characteristics:

Vacillation between choices; delayed decision making

- **Subjective Findings:** Verbalizes uncertainty and negative consequences of perceived alternatives; expresses distress related to advancing health problems and disabilities; discusses frustrations related to health care provider or family demands for decisions; examines personal values and beliefs related to quality and quantity of life; repeatedly asks for input and opinions

- **Objective Findings:** Physical signs of stress and tension; behaviors that are counter to expressed goals; unrealistic expectations; confusion; lack of information or previous experience with treatment regimens; delays decision making or chooses not to choose; vacillation between potential choices; seeks second and third opinions

Outcome Criteria:

Effective, informed decisions

Interventions	Rationales
Implement interventions discussed in Decisional Conflict in Secondary Prevention	Provides initial assessment and clarification processes for the client

Interventions	Rationales
Focus on end-of-life issues such as desires for continuing therapy, comfort and pain control, concerns about funeral plans, concerns about disposition of possessions, and care for survivors, especially children; determine presence of legal documents such as wills, living wills, powers of attorney, etc.; determine client desires; provide support for client decisions	Provides appropriate attention to the tasks of this phase of life; supports client's desires and decisions
Involve family and significant others as much as possible: determine their concerns; assess their willingness to support client's decisions; assist with conflict resolution; encourage focus on client needs for comfort and support through final life phases	Acknowledges importance of family and significant others in the dying process; provides support to them as they deal with loss and grief while continuing to support the client's wishes

Evaluation:

The client:

1. Receives support for end-of-life choices
2. Derives comfort from knowing that those decisions will be honored before, during, and after death

The family:

1. Is aware of the choices made by the client
2. Receives support to follow through on decisions
3. Experiences minimal discord during the dying and post-death periods

Altered Thought Process

A state in which the client experiences a disruption in cognitive operations and activities.

*Author's Note:

Cognitive and communications abilities decrease during the terminal phase as the client focus turns inward. This is especially distressing to the family and significant others who want their relationship with the client to continue on an interactive level. While safety issues are foremost for the client, the family will need emotional support.

Related to:

CNS infection with HIV, resulting in AIDS dementia complex (ADC); aseptic meningitis; opportunistic infections of the CNS; CNS malignancies; hypoxemia related to pulmonary disease; drug reactions; reactions to radiation therapy; depression or anxiety; fever; stress; substance use; fear; loss and grief; emotional trauma; isolation; unclear communication; dehydration and/or nutritional deficits; electrolyte or acid-base imbalances; sensory overload or deprivation; social isolation

Defining Characteristics:

Inaccurate interpretation of internal or external stimuli

- **Subjective Findings:** Client may not be able to provide subjective information

- **Objective Findings:** Disoriented to person, place, time; altered levels of consciousness; impaired memory; attention deficit; hyperactivity; inappropriate or fantasy-based thinking; disturbed thought flow; disturbed thought content; inappropriate affect; impaired problem solving; social withdrawal; behavior changes; signs of meningitis or other CNS disease; signs of self-neglect; sensory-perceptual deficits; coma

Outcome Criteria:

Physical safety maintained; family support provided

Interventions/Rationales

Initiate interventions described in Altered Thought Process in Tertiary Prevention; focus is now on client safety and support of family members and significant others.

Evaluation:

The client:

1. Remains safe without physical injury
2. Experiences the least possible effects of altered thought processes with minimal disorientation, confusion, anxiety, or other dementia symptoms

The family:

1. Assists in the continuing care of the client with a focus on physical safety
2. Receives physical and emotional support

Anxiety

A state in which the client experiences a vague, uneasy feeling in response to a nonspecific or unknown threat.

Related to:

Concerns about terminal care and pain control; unknowns related to death and dying; awareness of concerns and uneasiness among family and significant others

Defining Characteristics:

Stress manifested in physical, emotional, and cognitive symptoms

- **Subjective Findings:** Expresses fear, anger, denial, hostility, regret, helplessness, inability to sleep, concern over forgetfulness; makes statements about lack of confidence in abilities of caregivers; discusses apprehension, worry, nervousness, loneliness, concerns about death and/or life after death

- **Objective Findings:** Physiologic symptoms of stress, insomnia, fatigue, apprehension; helplessness; nervousness; tension; fear; irritability; anger; withdrawal; lack of initiative; decreased attention span; difficulty learning/remembering; decreased coping ability; avoidance mechanisms; decreased communication abilities; unrealistic expectations

Outcome Criteria:

Anxiety decreased to manageable levels

Interventions/Rationales

Initiate interventions described in Anxiety in Tertiary Prevention.

Evaluation:

The client:

1. Discusses concerns
2. Uses effective coping strategies to manage anxiety
3. Verbalizes a decrease in anxiety

Fatigue

A state in which the client feels an overwhelming and sustained sense of exhaustion and decreased ability to maintain usual levels of physical or mental effort.

*Author's Note:

Fatigue becomes more pronounced during the terminal phase of all diseases including AIDS. Clients will require more time for rest and sleep. Family members and significant others will need to learn about this increased need in order to provide appropriate support and to use periods of wakefulness for caring interactions.

Related to:

Advancing physical effects of HIV and opportunistic diseases; fever; weakness; neuromuscular changes; anemia; malnutrition; diarrhea; prolonged immobility; electrolyte imbalance; side effects of medications for pain and nausea; overwhelming emotional demands; depression; anxiety and stress; lack of social support

Defining Characteristics:

Overwhelming and persistent feelings of tiredness

- **Subjective Findings:** Client may not be able to provide subjective information

- **Objective Findings:** Prolonged periods of sleep; dyspnea on mild exertion; requires frequent rest periods; irritability; decreased ability to concentrate; lethargy; listlessness

Outcome Criteria:

Preservation and efficient use of energy

Interventions/Rationales

Initiate interventions discussed in Fatigue in Secondary Prevention; focus is now on providing for physical needs during prolonged periods of rest to prevent skin breakdown, respiratory distress, incontinence, and safety problems.

Evaluation:

The client:

1. Receives appropriate physical care as fatigue increases
2. Remains comfortable during periods of wakefulness

Fear

A state in which the client experiences a feeling of dread related to the prospect of death.

Related to:

Progression of symptoms of chronic HIV and opportunistic diseases; development of complications such as sensory impairment, physical disabilities, weight loss, cognitive impairment, pain; need for hospitalization, home care, invasive procedures, medications or radiation; loss or change in usual surroundings including significant others

Defining Characteristics:

Feelings of dread or apprehension

- **Subjective Findings:** Describes fearful situations; discusses worries about pain and death process; reports panic attacks or obsessions

- **Objective Findings:** Avoidance behaviors; attention, performance, or control deficits; behavioral manifestations of fear including crying, aggressive behaviors, hypervigilance, dysfunctional immobility, compulsive mannerisms, increased questioning; physical signs of fear including trembling, muscle tension, palpitations, tachycardia, increased blood pressure, shortness of breath, tachypnea, nausea and vomiting, anorexia, diarrhea, dry mouth, diaphoresis, dilated pupils; social paralysis; anger; grief

Outcome Criteria:

Fear reduced to a manageable level

Interventions/Rationales

Initiate interventions described in Fear in Secondary Prevention; focus is on providing for comfort and allaying fears related to the dying process and life after death; assistance should be solicited as acceptable to the client from family, significant others, and identified spiritual supports.

Evaluation:

The client:

1. Discusses fears about death and dying
2. Verbalizes decreased levels of fear

Hopelessness

A state in which the individual sees limited or no alternatives or personal choices available and is unable to mobilize energy on own behalf.

*Author's Note:

Hopelessness increases as physical and mental abilities deteriorate during the dying process. Frequently, there is no hope for survival and this leads to despair on the part of the client.

Related to:

Progression of HIV disease; failing or deteriorating physical condition; unexpected signs and symptoms; pain and discomfort; fatigue; impaired functions; social isolation; dependence; long-term stress; loss of spiritual belief system; prolonged activity restrictions

Defining Characteristics:

Apathy

- **Subjective Findings:** Expresses profound, overwhelming apathy; perceives deteriorating status as an impossible situation with no solutions; discusses desire to give up

- **Objective Findings:** Slowed responses; lack of energy; increased or decreased sleep; flat affect; decreased ability to solve problems and make decisions; unable to recognize solutions or sources of hope; anorexia and weight loss; severe depression; social withdrawal; anger; negative thought processes; confusion; poor communication skills; unrealistic perceptions; pessimism; suicidal ideation

Outcome Criteria:

Realistic goal setting

Interventions/Rationales

Initiate interventions described in Hopelessness in Secondary Prevention.

Evaluation:

The client:

1. Reconsiders personal life values and accomplishments
2. Reinforces positive relationships with significant others

Altered Family Processes

A state in which a family that normally functions effectively experiences a challenge to its functional status when a family member is faced with terminal HIV disease.

*Author's Note:

As HIV disease progresses, the family will often become more involved with health care and support. During the terminal phase, the client very often moves back home, either into a relative's home or at least to a nearby location, thus increasing the family's interactions and responsibilities. These activities and the impending death of the client add stress to the function of the family even if there is a well-established, loving relationship with the client. All families who are dealing with HIV disease need extra support and assistance.

Related to:

Terminal phases of HIV disease; observation of a family member who is dealing with pain, discomfort, and deterioration; disruption of family routines; change in family member's ability to function in established, comfortable manner; financial burdens on the family related to health care requirements and changes in employment or income; emotional changes as family member with HIV disease becomes more dependent; blame; guilt; fear; anger; grief

Defining Characteristics:

Family system does not adapt to changes

- **Subjective Findings:** *Family Member(s)* express feelings of anger, guilt, shame, rejection, fatigue, fear, anxiety, grief; discuss concerns about ability to continue support for client

- **Objective Findings:** Poor communication within family; physical, emotional, spiritual, or safety needs of individual not met by family; financial stressors; inability to adapt to health care requirements, especially hospitalization and home health care; inability to accept appropriate assistance; rigidity in roles and functions without demonstration of ability to adapt as HIV disease progresses

Outcome Criteria:

Maintenance of supportive family structure

Interventions/Rationales

Initiate interventions described in Altered Family Processes in Tertiary Prevention; focus is on assisting family to deal with increasing client care needs while also working through grief issues (see below).

Evaluation:

Family members:

1. Verbalize concerns about ability to provide care
2. Communicate concerns to other family members

3. Resolve issues through shared responsibilities
4. Maintain support system for all family members

Grieving

A state in which the client and family members experience a natural human response to loss.

Related to:

Progressive and terminal HIV disease; observations of increasing debility; loss of physical and mental abilities; weakness; fatigue

Defining Characteristics:

Physical and psychosocial reactions to loss

- **Subjective Findings:** *Client* focuses discussions on death and life after death or may not be able to discuss these issues; *Family Members* report concerns about ability to deal with death of client; verbalize feelings of guilt, anger, denial, despair, worthlessness, sorrow, anxiety, self-blame, loneliness, fatigue, helplessness, shock, yearning, numbness

- **Objective Findings:** *Family Members (especially primary caregiver)* show depressed affect; decreased ability/desire to communicate with others; fatigue; neglect of personal grooming, nutrition, and personal care needs

Outcome Criteria:

Integration of loss(es) into life; focus is on family members and significant others

Interventions	Rationales
Assist client and family members to discuss loss(es): help identify loss(es) that have been experienced; encourage discussions that help identify the personal meanings of each loss; allow expressions of emotions and feelings about the loss(es); ask about previous losses and previous coping methods; encourage discussion of fears related to each loss; allow for periods of silence and crying	Provides assessment information that will be used as a base to plan interventions; recognizes the importance of loss(es); establishes an open, trusting relationship in which frank discussions about loss and grief can occur; promotes self-reflection; focuses on client as well as family members and significant others
Identify usual coping mechanisms; reinforce healthy mechanisms such as talking to friends, exercising, meditating, etc.; refer to counseling for unhealthy responses such as drinking, drugging, acting-out sexually or physically, withdrawal	Reinforces healthy responses that have a history of success; circumvents return to less healthy coping mechanisms

Interventions	Rationales	Interventions	Rationales
Explain grief reactions that frequently occur (shock, denial, disbelief, isolation; bargaining; depression; acceptance; physical responses); explain that each individual works through losses in a unique way and that the client and/or family will not necessarily progress in any set pattern	Establishes a knowledge base; allows client/family member to progress as needed without feeling the need to meet goals and stages	*Depression:* acknowledge grief and promote sharing of feelings about loss; assess level of depression and provide appropriate interventions related to suicide prevention and/or consultations with mental health professionals	
Provide support to work through grief reaction; explain need for various reactions; promote grief work	Supports individual with specific interventions at each phase of the grief reaction	*Anger:* encourage verbalizations about anger; support others who may be the focus of anger; encourage identification of appropriate target for anger and discuss issues important to specific problem	
Denial: do not push movement past denial before emotionally capable; observe and prevent potentially dangerous activities that may occur as a result of denial		*Guilt:* encourage discussions about feelings related to guilt; help identify reality related to the loss; refrain from buying into a system of "shoulds" and "should nots," return instead to a reality-based discussion	
Isolation/Rejection of Others: allow privacy; explain need for solitude; encourage gradual increases in amount of social interaction		*Fear:* maintain safe environment for discussions	

Interventions	Rationales
Identify and refer to resources that will support grief work (mental health counselors, support groups, spiritual leaders, etc.); refer to resources; help establish contact with desired support systems	Provides long-term support for the grieving process

Evaluation:

The client:

1. Receives support needed to progress through dying process
2. Receives needed physical care

Family members:

1. Express grief and, in the process, discover meanings of loss and coping methods
2. Begin to cope with losses
3. Maintain social contact with supportive significant others

Dysfunctional Grieving

A state in which the individual suffers a prolonged response to grief that is unresolved and detrimental.

*Author's Note:

Family and significant others may suffer the effects of dysfunctional grieving prior to or following the death of a loved one. Many families have dealt with the stigma and discrimination related to HIV infection and AIDS by hiding the diagnosis behind other conditions such as pneumonia or cancer. Families who choose this tactic may have additional troubles with the grief process because of the subterfuge and inability to confide in usual social or spiritual support systems. Some family members may not have been able to resolve issues related to the client's lifestyle or infection; those individuals may have to deal with overwhelming guilt and denial as well as grief. More and more families are experiencing multiple losses as HIV expresses itself as a family disease. In these cases there may not be adequate time to grieve between losses or the number of deaths may cause an emotional state of numbness. Other survivors simply may not be able to deal with the loss through healthy grief processes. Continuing support of the family and significant others is an important part of care in the terminal phase of AIDS. Unfortunately, survivors often lose access to the health care system that has supported them through the life and death of their loved one. Health care providers who never knew the deceased may be required to step in to fill the void created after the client's death.

Related to:

Negation of loss by others; social isolation; assuming the role of "the strong one"; inability to attend to grieving because of problems associated with unresolved psychosocial and financial problems; fear of the mourning process

Defining Characteristics:

Prolonged or delayed reactions to loss

- **Subjective Findings:** *Family Members* or *Significant Others* report problems with concentration, developing new interests, low self-esteem, eating, sleeping, activity, and libido levels; discuss feelings of despair and hopelessness

- **Objective Findings:** Inhibition, suppression or absence of emotional reactions to loss; prolonged denial of loss; decreased participation in formerly helpful spiritual activities; hopelessness; suicidal ideation; somatic expressions of fear such as hyperventilation, choking, dyspnea; social isolation or withdrawal; fails to restructure life after loss

Outcome Criteria:

Progressive resolution of grief

Interventions	Rationales
Determine if individual is "stuck" in a particular phase or with a particular emotional grief response; develop specific interventions to cope with these specific problems; also see Decisional Conflict, Anxiety, Fear, Hopelessness, Powerlessness, Grieving (above), and Ineffective Individual Coping, Ineffective Denial (below)	Focuses interventions on identified area of need
Assist with identifying and developing interventions for problems that can increase, delay, or prolong grief	Numerous problems can impact on the grief process and must be considered

Interventions	Rationales
Help individual acknowledge awareness of loss: provide opportunities to discuss loss; restate reality in nonthreatening manner; present factual information; do not argue about reality of loss; use guided imagery or role playing to allow confrontation of loss	Promotes recognition of loss as meaningful; initiates recognition of need to grieve
Promote adaptation to loss: facilitate contact with others who have experienced similar losses; encourage use of previously helpful (and healthy) coping mechanisms; provide consistent and correct information, clarify misconceptions, correct misinformation; offer hope for successful adaptation; encourage time for rest, relaxation, exercise, and nutrition; provide contacts with mental health professionals, religious/spiritual leaders, family, and friends who are acceptable supports	Encourages positive activities that can move individual through grief process; decreases knowledge deficits; acknowledges need for "time off" to replenish energy stores; promotes social interactions for support

Evaluation:

The family member or significant other:

1. Acknowledges personal meaning of loss
2. Initiates efforts to deal with loss
3. Reports decreasing discomfort related to grief
4. Moves into grief work process

Parental Role Conflict

A state in which a parent experiences role conflict in response to his/her own terminal state caused by HIV infection.

Related to:

Parent's terminal state; decreased parental role; multiple health care providers in the home; hospitalization of the parent; multiple family stressors; financial problems; inadequate social supports; single parents who provide sole support for children; disruption of family routines; health care system that does not consider family cultural, social, and childrearing norms

Defining Characteristics:

Children without parental support

- **Subjective Findings:** *Parent* expresses concerns about continued care for child(ren); verbalizes feelings of guilt, fear, anger, anxiety, frustration, or inadequacy in relation to child care

- **Objective Findings:** *Children* demonstrate poor nutrition and hygiene, lack of parental control in social and academic activities, and/or clinging behaviors, fear, anxiety, depression, guilt, anger; older children may have taken over parental roles, especially in a single-parent family; *Parent* displays evidence of stress, fear, anxiety, guilt, fatigue, depression, or anger

Outcome Criteria:

Family receives support required to maintain appropriate support of children

Interventions	Rationales
Initiate interventions discussed in Parental Role Conflict in Tertiary Prevention	Provides assessment and initial interventions that can assist the family to remain intact while preparing for continuing child care in emergencies and after client's death
Support children: encourage expressions of fear, hope, concern, grief, anger, and guilt; discuss issues related to HIV infection, illness, pain, death, and dying as requested by each child in an age appropriate manner; encourage parent(s) to include children in plans for the future, asking for their assistance and consent in choosing guardians and living conditions after the parent's death, for example; refer to child mental health providers for counseling during the course of anticipated and final losses	Identifies problems presented by each child; initiates interactions to assist the child to deal with the loss of one or more parents; encourages child to express concerns and feelings in a supportive atmosphere

Evaluation:

The parent:

1. Continues to provide support for children
2. Identifies and takes steps to plan for and/or rectify problems
3. Verbalizes decreased stress and anxiety related to providing long-term support for children

The children:

1. Identify resources and sources of support for times of crisis
2. Maintain a positive relationship with the parent
3. Demonstrate decreasing levels of anxiety, fear, anger, and/or acting-out behaviors
4. Receive supportive services to prepare for loss and to work through grief

Impaired Social Interaction

A state in which an individual experiences negative, insufficient, or unsatisfactory responses from social interactions.

Related to:

Terminal phase of HIV disease; loss of body function; hearing or visual deficits; fatigue; severe anxiety; hopelessness; powerlessness; lack of self-care skills; depression; social isolation; need for hospitalization or home care; limited physical mobility; self-concept disturbance; altered thought processes; lack of available significant others/friends; communication barriers

Defining Characteristics:

Lack of stable, supportive relationships

- **Subjective Findings:** Reports unsatisfactory interactions with family and peers; discusses need for support from others; blames others for interpersonal problems; discusses feelings of regret and remorse

- **Objective Findings:** Unable to receive or communicate a sense of belonging, caring, or interest in others; uses unsuccessful or inappropriate social behaviors; exhibits dependent behaviors; unaware of how s/he is perceived by others; *Family* reports changes in interactions with client

Outcome Criteria:

Improved ability to relate to others

Interventions	Rationales
Develop an individual and supportive relationship with the client	Develops a trusting relationship with the nurse in order for interventions to progress; in some cases health care providers may be the client's only continuing social support
Help client identify family members and significant others who need to be informed of her or his terminal state; with client permission, initiate contact with these individuals	Some clients have alienated important social supports, others have made a conscious decision to keep their physical condition a secret, and there are those who have been abandoned by their loved ones; terminal illness may cause the client and/or family and significant others to seek reconciliation

Interventions	Rationales
Provide continuing support to client as well as to family members and significant others who decide to re-establish contact during the terminal phase; refer to counseling services as needed	Acknowledges the difficulty of these situations; some reconciliations are gratifying while others are disruptive
Refer to community support systems as appropriate such as HIV service organizations, mental health and family counseling, social services	Provides continuing support; assists client to cope with problems related to impaired or absent social interactions

Evaluation:

The client:

1. Receives supportive care during terminal processes
2. Has an opportunity to reconcile with significant others prior to death

Social Isolation

A state in which the client and/or family experiences aloneness that is perceived to be negative or threatening and to have been imposed by others.

Related to:

Stigma associated with HIV infection, disability, disfigurement, dying, death, sexual orientation, and/or substance use; social fears related to communicable nature of HIV infection; rejection by family, friends, neighbors; withdrawal from people and activities; sensory-perceptual deficits; altered thought processes; extreme anxiety; depression; poverty; need for hospitalization or home health care; alienation; low self-esteem; geographic distance from family; impaired mobility; body image disturbance; inadequate personal resources

Defining Characteristics:

Isolation from society

- **Subjective Findings:** *Client, Family,* and/or *Significant Others* express feelings of loneliness, isolation, uselessness, hopelessness, depression, lack of purpose, rejection; state perception that isolation has been imposed by others; verbalize desire for more human contact; report multiple losses, barriers to social contact, changes in living arrangements, or inadequate social support system; acknowledge inability to concentrate and make decisions; describe changes in sleeping or eating patterns

- **Objective Findings:** Increasing evidence of physical or mental deterioration; depression, anxiety, or anger; failure to interact with others; aggressive or hostile behaviors; absence of supportive others, lack of visitors; withdrawal; inability or refusal to communicate; exhaustion; single-minded focus on care for client

Outcome Criteria:

Maintenance of social relationships or adaptation to changes in relationships

Interventions	Rationales
Initiate interventions discussed in Impaired Social Interaction in Tertiary Prevention	Assesses state of social isolation; suggests interventions to alleviate problems associated with isolation
With client's permission, encourage interactions with family and significant others by instructing others in mechanisms of HIV transmission and prevention of transmission; involving them in providing care; encouraging communications through letters and telephone calls	Supports continuing efforts of significant others to be involved in client's life; reassures others about risk of infection; provides positive environment for social interaction
Spend social time with family and significant others when treatments and physical care are not required; interact in a social manner by discussing topics of interest that are not necessarily related to HIV disease, death, dying, or survivor concerns; use touch as acceptable	Expresses unconditional regard that extends beyond providing care for the client; models social interaction skills; provides human contact

Interventions	Rationales
Assist others to develop plans for expanding social interactions: identify activities that interest them; provide resources for social interaction in the community (support groups, initiating telephone contact with significant others, etc.); promote realistic course of action that does not overburden the family caregiver; identify potential barriers to social contacts and develop means to overcome the barriers; provide respite care so that family caregivers can spend time in social or relaxation activities	Provides opportunities to increase social interactions; encourages planning to circumvent barriers prior to their development

Evaluation:

The family/significant other:

1. Maintains important social contacts through the process of losing a loved one
2. Receives social support as needed
3. Uses social supports to help cope with the difficulties of client care, deterioration, and loss

Altered Sexuality Patterns

A state in which an individual or partner expresses concerns about the client's sexuality as it is affected by advancing HIV disease.

*Author's Note:

Terminal disease is a great inhibitor of sexual intercourse. It is important to remember, however, that sexuality encompasses more than sexual intercourse. Sometimes the primary need is to have the feeling of attachment and personal touch that can only be provided by an emotionally attached significant sexual other. This is especially true as the individual feels the attachments to life slipping away.

Related to:

Progressing disability, fatigue, and lack of energy; pain; side effects of medications; altered self-concept and/or body image disturbance; self-esteem problems; loss of sexual partner through death or abandonment; lack of privacy; presence of stressors related to health care, finances, depression, anxiety, guilt, negative social attitude toward sexual activity in terminal individuals; lack of information about alternative means of sexual expression; social isolation; decreased sex drive

Defining Characteristics:

Concern over the loss of intimate contact

- **Subjective Findings:** Expresses concern about intimacy; verbalizes guilt, shame, or stigma associated with continuing desire for intimacy; discusses frustrations; expresses concerns about loss of appearance or function that could decrease partner's desire for intimate contact

- **Objective Findings:** Reluctance to discuss issues related to intimacy; guilt; fear; shame

Outcome Criteria:

Maintenance of intimacy with significant other

Interventions	Rationales
Discuss issues of intimacy with client and his/her significant other	Opens topic for discussion; assesses problems, doubts, and concerns
Provide information to the significant other about safety, continuing needs for intimacy, and changes in intimacy needs; explain that, at this time, sexual intercourse is less of a priority while intimate touch and holding are more important; encourage significant other to talk to the client in a manner that reinforces the established intimacy	Provides information to allay fears; provides social support for continued intimacy and support of client; assists significant other to fulfill personal needs for intimacy as s/he prepares for the loss of a loved one
Provide privacy for client and significant other for periods of intimate exchanges	Decreases inhibitions; provides a more usual atmosphere for intimate contacts

Evaluation:

The client:

1. Receives the benefit of continuing intimacy
2. Maintains intimate contact with significant other during dying processes

The significant other:

1. Receives the benefit of continuing intimacy
2. Maintains intimate contact with client during dying processes
3. Initiates healthy grief process prior to and after the death of the client

Caregiver Role Strain

A state in which a caregiver (other than a professional health care provider) experiences physical, emotional, economic, or social difficulty in performing the caregiver role.

Related to:

Terminal state of the client and his or her increased care needs; conflicting role demands of the caregiver (i.e., career, child care, responsibilities to other members of the family, etc.); impaired health status of the caregiver; caregiver's lack of experience in providing health care, especially during terminal phases of a disease; history of familial dysfunction or poor caregiver-care receiver relationship; caregiver's lack of coping patterns; need for direct, long-term, 24 hour care in the home; care receiver develops psychological, cognitive, sensory-perceptual problems; care receiver develops bizarre behaviors, becomes incontinent, or manifests signs of dementia; relative difficulty of required health care interventions; caregiver apprehension related to ability to provide care; caregiver experiences or anticipates multiple losses related to relationship with care receiver, career, finances, social system, etc.; caregiver's feelings of depression, anxiety, anger, guilt; caregiver and/or care receiver has unrealistic expectations; caregiver experiences isolation as well as insufficient rest, relaxation, respite, finances

Defining Characteristics:

Decreased ability to provide care

- **Subjective Findings:** *Caregiver* reports feeling exhausted; discusses declining health status; verbalizes feelings of depression, loss, grief, stress, anxiety, sleep pattern disturbances, poor self-concept; relates emotional response to changes in expected relationship (i.e., son is supposed to care for mother in her old age instead of her caring for him in a terminal disease, partner/spouse expected a sharing of life burdens, children want to depend on parent for support, etc.); discusses family/role conflicts related to caregiving role; describes withdrawal from social contacts and usual leisure activities due to fatigue, sense of responsibility, fear of stigma or discrimination

- **Objective Findings:** *Caregiver* is unable to complete required tasks; declining health; emotional liability; social withdrawal; refuses to allow others to provide respite care; insists on providing 24 hour care; becomes preoccupied with caregiving routine; apprehensive; anxious; angry; depressed

Outcome Criteria:

Effective support for caregiver

Interventions/Rationales

Initiate interventions described in Caregiver Role Strain in Tertiary Prevention.

Evaluation:

The caregiver:

1. Provides safe, supportive care to the HIV-infected client

2. Acknowledges need for personal support and accesses resources in family and community

3. Shares frustrations about difficulty of care for significant other

4. Receives assistance from family members and/or professional caregivers

Ineffective Individual Coping

A state in which an individual experiences difficulties in meeting life's demands because of an impairment of adaptive and problem-solving abilities.

Related to:

Terminal HIV disease and associated physical and psychosocial disturbances; disruptions of relationships; poverty; inadequate support system; lack of resources; low self-esteem; perceived lack of control; stress overload; multiple losses; pain; hopelessness; powerlessness; loss of hope and/or spiritual values; social withdrawal

Defining Characteristics:

Ineffective coping

- **Subjective Findings:** *Client* may not be able to provide subjective information, or may verbalize fears of becoming dependent or not having acceptable care available as illness and disability increase

- **Objective Findings:** Inability to meet basic needs; inability to identify or access resources; low morale; hopelessness; social withdrawal; inflexible; hypervigilant; refuses assistance; does not maintain personal hygiene or ADLs

Outcome Criteria:

Receives needed assistance during terminal disease

Interventions	Rationales
Assess care situation: Is client receiving appropriate care? Who is providing care for the client? Is situation acceptable to the client? to the caregiver?	Provides basic information for use in developing interventions

Interventions	Rationales
Discuss various care options with the client and/or family and significant others (professional home care, home care by family or significant others, hospice, long-term care facilities, acute care facilities, etc.); determine client desires and appropriateness of those desires; discuss problems if desires cannot be safely carried out and assist with developing alternative plans; refer to case management, social services, or specific facilities to initiate selected care options	Maintains client input as possible; assures care in an appropriate and safe environment; supports family and significant other input

Evaluation:

The client:

1. Accepts support from nursing relationship and other resources
2. Receives necessary care during terminal phases of HIV disease

Ineffective Denial

A state in which the client and/or family and significant others consciously or unconsciously attempt to disavow the terminal aspect of HIV disease in order to reduce anxiety or fear. The denial usually results in a detrimental effect on the client's physical, mental, or social status.

Related to:

Inability to acknowledge terminal disease; inability to acknowledge that one's life is ending; inability to acknowledge impending loss of a loved one; multiple losses

Defining Characteristics:

Inability to accept terminal status

- **Subjective Findings:** *Client, Family,* and/or *Significant Others* deny that increasing symptoms are relevant, serious or dangerous; deny or cannot admit that advancing symptoms have an impact on capabilities and/or life pattern; dismiss importance of distressing symptoms or events; express feelings of inadequacy, guilt, loneliness, despair, fear, anxiety, stress, anger, frustration

- **Objective Findings:** *Client* refuses to acknowledge decreasing abilities and state of health; attempts to continue in usual routines resulting in fatigue, dyspnea, depression, and frustration; refuses to discuss plans for survivors; expresses anger and defensiveness when issues such as increased need for health care are mentioned; *Family* and *Significant Others* refuse to discuss issues related to death, funeral plans, survivor plans, or need for increased care; will not allow client to discuss these issues; promote hope in futile situations; insist that client continue usual routines and activities

Outcome Criteria:

Acceptance of terminal disease

Interventions/Rationales

Initiate interventions described in Ineffective Denial in Tertiary Prevention; focus is on assisting client and family members to accept and plan for care during terminal phases of disease without making them lose hope.

Evaluation:

The client:

1. Maintains supportive relationship with nurse and family caregivers
2. Experiences reduction in fear and/or anxiety

The family/significant other:

1. Develops a realistic appraisal of the client's health status
2. Provides support and comfort to the client during the dying process
3. Discusses concerns and fears related to the impending loss of a loved one

Ineffective Family Coping: Disabling

A state in which a family demonstrates destructive behaviors that disable the ability to adapt to the health challenge created by terminal HIV disease in one of the family members.

Related to:

Families with a history of dysfunction, abuse, substance use, emotional disturbance, or poor coping abilities; families that are unwilling or unable to meet psychosocial needs of their members; terminal disease and related care needs; decreasing ability of family member with HIV disease to care for self, contribute to family support, or maintain usual roles; unrealistic expectations of ability to provide support or continue responsibilities; anxiety; fear of stigma associated with HIV infection and social discrimination; lack of support from extended family, social networks, religious affiliations, etc.; ambivalent family relationships related to sexual orientation or drug use issues; multiple stressors and losses; refusal to access assistance from external resources; presence of an authoritarian family member; familial isolation; knowledge deficits

Defining Characteristics:

Ineffective family processes

- **Subjective Findings:** *Client* complains about neglect, abuse, indifference, rejection, intolerance, violence, or abandonment from family; develops helplessness and dependence; expresses concerns about family's ability to cope; *Family Member(s)* observe and report neglect, abuse, indifference, rejection, intolerance, violence, or abandonment toward client; report anxiety, depression, powerlessness, hopelessness, guilt, denial, anger, fear, blame, rejection, jealousy, agitation, hostility, aggression, inability to cope; over or underestimate capabilities of client and distort realities of the situation; take on symptoms of HIV

- **Objective Findings:** *Family Members* do not maintain contact as evidenced by a lack of visits, telephone calls, letters, etc.; inadequate care or support for HIV-infected client in home care situations; neglect; desertion; actions that are detrimental to client's physical, psychosocial, economic, and/or health care status; demeaning remarks directed toward client; actions that promote dependence, low self-esteem, and helplessness in client; inadequate or unhealthy coping behaviors such as denial, abuse, increased substance use, etc.; lack of any signs of a meaningful or supportive family environment; inadequate knowledge and skills to provide care or support

Outcome Criteria:

Effective family coping; appropriate care and support for client during terminal phase

Interventions/Rationales

Initiate interventions described in Ineffective Family Coping: Disabling in Tertiary Prevention.

Evaluation:

The client:

1. Receives needed care and support during terminal phase

The family:

1. Interacts in a supportive and caring manner
2. Demonstrates ability to provide care within limits specified by group consensus
3. Accesses and accepts available resources that promote ability to provide continued support and care to all family members

Relocation Stress Syndrome

A state in which the client suffers physical and/or psychosocial disturbance as a result of a transfer from one environment to another.

*Author's Note:

Terminal disease frequently necessitates a move to an environment that will allow continuous care. For clients with terminal HIV disease, care locations can include acute care hospitals, hospice centers, long-term care facilities, or a home setting with professional or family/friend/significant other support. Many clients with terminal HIV disease choose to die at home. This is only possible, however, if adequate care is available for the client. Often this means leaving an independent living situation and moving into the home of a relative or friend. This creates significant upheaval for all those involved.

Related to:

Terminal status; decreasing physical health and functioning; need for hospitalization or increased assistance in the home; decreased control in living arrangements; major differences between old and new environments; changes in levels of care; multiple losses experienced prior to and during relocation; abandonment requiring changes in environment in order to receive needed physical, social, and economic supports; lack of preparation or control of relocation

Defining Characteristics:

Acute stress related to relocation

- **Subjective Findings:** Verbalizes stress, discomfort, reluctance, insecurity, anger, anxiety, grief, and feelings of displacement; expresses feelings of increased dependency, loneliness, loss of identity, powerlessness, and uncertainty about the future; increases demands on family and caregivers; makes unfavorable comparisons between old and new environments

- **Objective Findings:** Changes in sleep and eating patterns; increasing dependence, questioning, and distrusting behaviors; restlessness; sad affect; aggressive behaviors; confusion and disorientation; withdrawal and detachment; withholds self from social interaction and attachment

Outcome Criteria:

Appropriate grief for losses and adjustment to new environment

Interventions/Rationales

Initiate interventions discussed in Relocation Stress Syndrome in Tertiary Prevention; focus is on helping all affected individuals to cope with new stressors and to support grieving process.

Evaluation:

The client:

1. Acknowledges need for relocation
2. Takes an active part in planning for changes
3. Discusses concerns and grieves for losses
4. Becomes comfortable in new environment

Spiritual Distress

A state of disruption in the individual's belief or value system that provides strength, hope, and meaning to life, and that transcends the individual's biological and psychosocial nature.

Related to:

Terminal HIV disease; multiple losses; pain; disability; social stigma; social isolation; feelings that spiritual system has failed; lack of previously developed spiritual values; denial of need for spirituality; separation from religious, cultural, or family ties; admission to a facility that prevents practice of spiritual rituals that require privacy, special diets, freedom from interruption, etc.

Defining Characteristics:

Searching for a spiritual base

- **Subjective Findings:** Questions belief system, relationship with higher power, personal significance, need for suffering; expresses ambivalence about beliefs; describes a sense of spiritual emptiness; initiates discussions about meaning of life, death, disease; relates history of negative response from religious leaders or congregations; expresses anger toward God

- **Objective Findings:** Requests spiritual assistance; appetite and sleep disturbances; crying

Outcome Criteria:

Receives spiritual support and comfort

Interventions/Rationales

Initiate interventions described in Spiritual Distress in Secondary Prevention.

Evaluation:

The client:

1. Continues and/or enhances positive spiritual practices
2. Explores options for spiritual development and support
3. Expresses satisfaction with belief system and associated supports
4. Experiences enhanced inner peace and decreased somatic and emotional distress

Appendix I

Abbreviations Used in this Book

3TC - lamivudine (Epivir™)

ABGs - arterial blood gases

ACTG - AIDS Clinical Trials Group

ADC - AIDS dementia complex

ADLs - activities of daily living

AIDS - acquired immunodeficiency syndrome

ARC - AIDS related complex

ART - antiretroviral therapy

AZT - former name for zidovudine (Retrovir™, ZDV)

b.i.d. - twice a day

BSI - body substance isolation

BUN - blood urea nitrogen

CBC - complete blood count

CDC - Centers for Disease Control and Prevention

CMV - cytomegalovirus

CNS - central nervous system

CSF - cerebrospinal fluid

CT - computerized tomography

CXR - chest x-ray

d4T - stavudine (Zerit™)

ddC - zalcitabine (HIVID™)

ddI - didanosine (Videx™)

EIA/ELISA - enzyme linked immunoassay; a screening test for HIV antibody

FDC - follicular dendritic cell

GI - gastrointestinal

HBV - hepatitis B virus

HIV - human immunodeficiency virus

HSV - herpes simplex virus

IDV - indinavir (Crixivan™)

IFA - immunoflorescent assay; a confirming test for HIV antibodies

INH - isoniazid

KS - Kaposi's sarcoma

MAC - *Mycobacterium avium* complex

mm^3 - millimeter cubed

MRI - magnetic resonance imaging

MSM - men who have sex with men

NANDA - North American Nursing Diagnosis Association

NNRTI - non-nucleoside reverse transcriptase inhibitor

NRTI - nucleoside reverse transcriptase inhibitor

N/SEP - needle/syringe exchange program

OI - opportunistic infection

OSHA - Occupational Health and Safety
    Administration

PCP - *Pneumocystis carinii* pneumonia

PCR - polymerase chain reaction

PEP - post-exposure prophylaxis

PGL - persistent generalized
    lymphadenopathy

PI - protease inhibitor

PID - pelvic inflammatory disease

PML - progressive multifocal
    encephalopathy

PMS - pre-menstrual syndrome

PPD - purified protein derivative

PRN - as needed/when needed

q - every (as in every 8 hours - q8h)

qd - every day

RDA - recommended daily allowance

STD - sexually transmitted disease

t.i.d. - three times a day

TPM-SMX - trimethoprim-sulfamethoxazole

UP - universal precautions

VZIG - varicella zoster immune globulin

VZV - varicella zoster virus

WB - Western blot; a confirming test for
    HIV antibodies

ZDV - zidovudine (Retrovir™)

Appendix II

Resources

The Association of Nurses in AIDS Care (ANAC)

The Association of Nurses in AIDS Care is a professional organization made up of nurses and others who work or have an interest in any area of the HIV epidemic. The association publishes a bi-monthly newsletter and a bi-monthly journal (*The Journal of the Association of Nurses in AIDS Care*). ANAC sponsors an annual conference as well as other educational programs, and is an excellent source for educational, policy, and other professional resources. You can contact the ANAC national offices at:

Association of Nurses in AIDS Care
11250 Roger Bacon Drive, Suite 8
Reston, VA 20190-5202
1-800-260-6780 or 1-703-925-0081
1-703-435-4390
e-mail: AIDSNURSES@aol.com
website: http://www.anacnet.org/aids/

AIDS Education and Training Centers (ETCs)

The AIDS Education and Training Centers are a group of federally funded programs whose goals are to provide education about HIV infection and AIDS to health care providers in the United States. The ETCs are specifically charged to provide this education to nurses and nurse practitioners. Each state is covered by an existing ETC. Regional ETCs are listed below.

National Offices
AIDS ETC Program
Bureau of Health Professions
Parklawn Building, Room 9A-39
5600 Fishers Lane
Rockville, MD 20857
(301) 443-6560

Serving Nevada, Arizona, Hawaii, California
Pacific AIDS ETC
Department of Family & Community
  Medicine
500 Parnassus Ave., MU-3 East Box 0900
University of California
San Francisco, CA 94142-0900
(415) 502-8196

Serving Washington, Alaska, Montana, Idaho, Oregon
Northwest AIDS ETC
University of Washington
1001 Broadway, Suite 217, Box 359932
Seattle, WA 98122
(206) 221-4944

Serving Ohio, Michigan, Kentucky, Tennessee
Great Lakes/Tennessee Valley AIDS ETC
Wayne State University
2727 Second Avenue, Suite 142
Detroit, MI 48201
(313) 962-2000

Serving New York and the Virgin Islands
New York/Virgin Islands AIDS ETC
Columbia University School of Public Health
600 West 168th Street, 7th floor
New York, NY 10032
(212) 740-7292

Serving Puerto Rico
Puerto Rico AIDS ETC
University of Puerto Rico Medical Sciences
  Campus
GPO 36-5067 Room A-956
San Juan, PR 00936-5067
(787) 759-6528

Serving Connecticut, Maine, Massachusetts, New Hampshire, Rhode Island, Vermont
New England AIDS ETC
320 Washington Street, 3rd floor
Brookline, MA 02146
(617) 566-2283

Serving Alabama, Georgia, North Carolina, South Carolina
Southeast AIDS ETC
Emory University School of Medicine
Department of Family and Preventive
   Medicine
735 Gatewood Road, NE
Atlanta, GA 30322-4850
(404) 727-2929

Serving Arkansas, Louisiana, Mississippi
Delta Regional AIDS ETC
Louisiana State University Medical Center
136 South Roman Street, 3rd floor
New Orleans, LA 70112
(504) 568-3855

Serving North Dakota, South Dakota, Utah, Colorado, New Mexico, Nebraska, Kansas, Wyoming
Mountain-Plains Regional AIDS ETC
University of Colorado Health Science
   Center
4200 E. Ninth Ave., Box A-096
Denver, CO 80262
(303) 315-2516

Serving Iowa, Minnesota, Wisconsin, Illinois, Indiana, Missouri
Midwest AIDS Training & Education Center
University of Illinois at Chicago (M/C 779)
808 S. Wood St., Room 173
Chicago, IL 60612-7303
(312) 996-1364

Serving Pennsylvania
Pennsylvania AIDS ETC
University of Pittsburgh Graduate School of
   Public Health
130 DeSoto Street G-15 Parran Hall
Pittsburgh, PA 15261
(412) 624-1895

Serving Florida
Florida AIDS ETC Network
University of Miami School of Medicine
Department of Family Medicine &
   Community Health
600 Alton Road, Suite 502
Miami Beach, FL 33139
(305) 243-2846

Serving Maryland, District of Columbia, Virginia, West Virginia, Delaware
Mid-Atlantic AIDS ETC
Virginia Commonwealth University
P.O. Box 980159
Richmond, VA 23298-0159
(804) 828-2447

Serving Texas and Oklahoma
AIDS ETC for Texas and Oklahoma
University of Texas
1200 Herman Pressler St.
POB 20186
Houston, TX 77225
(713) 500-9205

Serving New Jersey
New Jersey AIDS ETC
University of Medicine and Dentistry of
   New Jersey
Center for Continuing Education
30 Bergen Street, ADMC #710
Newark, NJ 07107-3000
(973) 972-3690

Helpful WebSites:

Center for AIDS Prevention Studies -
   http://www.chanane.ucsf.edu/capsweb
CDC HIV/AIDS Prevention -
   http://www.cdc.gov/nchstp/hiv_aids/
   dhap.htm
HIV/AIDS Treatment Information Service -
   http://www.hivatis.org
HIV Information Web -
   http://www.jri.org/infoweb
National AIDS Clearinghouse -
   http://www.cdcnac.org

References

The Americans with Disabilities Act. (1992 & 1994). 42 U.S.C. s. 1201 et seq.

Anastasi, J.K., & Lee, V.S. (1994). HIV wasting: How to stop the cycle. *American Journal of Nursing*. 94(6), 18-24.

Antiviral briefs: ZDV reduces maternal transmission. (1994). *AIDS Patient Care*, 8, 164.

Bartlett, J.G. (1996). *Medical management of HIV infection* (Rev. ed.). Glenview, IL: Physicians and Scientists Publishing Co., Inc.

Bartlett, J.G. (1998). *Medical management of HIV infection* (Rev. ed.) Baltimore, MD: Johns Hopkins University, Department of Infectious Diseases.

Brennan, C., & Porche, D.J. (1997). HIV immunopathology. *Journal of the Association of Nurses in AIDS Care*, 8, 7-22.

Britten, N. (1994). Patients' ideas about medicines: A qualitative study in a general practice population. *British Journal of General Practice*, 44(387), 465-468.

Bradley-Springer, L. (1994). Reproductive decision making in the age of AIDS. *Image*, 26 (3), 241-246.

Bradley-Springer, L. (1996). Patient education for behavior change: Help from the transtheoretical and harm reduction models. *Journal of the Association of Nurses in AIDS Care*, 7, 23-33.

Bradley-Springer, L. (1997a). Needle and syringe exchange: Pride and prejudice. *Journal of the Association of Nurses AIDS Care*, 8, 3-5.

Bradley-Springer, L. (1997b). Prevention vs. treatment: An ongoing dilemma. *Journal of the Association of Nurses AIDS in Care*, 8, 87-88,94.

Bradley-Springer, L., & Fendrick, R. (1994). *HIV instant instructor cards*. El Paso: Skidmore- Roth Publishing.

Caldwell, M. (1993, August). The long shot. *Discover*, pp. 61-69.

Carey, R.F., Herman, W.A., Retta, S.M., Rinaldi, J.E., Herman, B.A., & Athey, T.W. (1992). Effectiveness of latex condoms as a barrier to human immunodeficiency virussized particles under conditions of simulated use. *Sexually Transmitted Diseases*, 19(4), 230-234.

Carpenito, L.J. (1993). *Handbook of nursing diagnosis* (5th ed.). Philadelphia: J.B. Lippincott.

Casey, K.M. (1995). Pathophysiology of HIV-1, clinical course, and treatment. In J.H. Flaskerud & P.J. Ungvarski (Eds.), *HIV/AIDS: A guide to nursing care* (3rd ed.). Philadelphia: Saunders.

Casey, K.M., Cohen, F., & Hughes, A.M. (Eds.). (1996). *ANAC's core curriculum for HIV/AIDS nursing*. Philadelphia: Nursecom.

Centers for Disease Control and Prevention (CDC). (1992, December 18). Recommendations and Reports: 1993 revised classification system for HIV infection and expanded surveillance case definition for AIDS among adolescents and adults. *Morbidity and Mortality Weekly Report*, 41 (RR-17), 1-17.

Centers for Disease Control and Prevention (CDC). (1994, August 5). Recommendations of the US Public Health Service Task Force on the use of zidovudine to reduce perinatal transmission of human immunodeficiency virus. *Morbidity and Mortality Weekly Report, 43*(RR-11), 1-20.

Centers for Disease Control and Prevention (CDC). (1996). Update: Provisional public health service recommendations for chemoprophylaxis after occupational exposure to HIV. *Morbidity and Mortality Weekly Report, 45*, 468-472.

Centers for Disease Control and Prevention (CDC). (1998). *HIV/AIDS surveillance report, 9*(2), 1-43.

Centers for Disease Control and Prevention (CDC) (1997). Recommendations and reports: 1997 USPHS/IDSA guidelines for the prevention of opportunistic infections in persons infected with human immunodeficiency virus. *Morbidity and Mortality Weekly Report, 46* (RR-12), 1-46.

Crespo-Fierro, M. (1997). Compliance/adherence and care management in HIV disease. *Journal of the Association of Nurses in AIDS Care, 8*(4), 43-54.

Daly, J.M. (1993). *NIC interventions linked to NANDA diagnoses.* Iowa City: Iowa Intervention project Research Team, University of Iowa.

de Vincenzi, I. (1994). A longitudinal study of human immunodeficiency virus transmission by heterosexual partners. *New England Journal of Medicine, 331*(6), 341-346.

Des Jarlais, D.C., Friedman, S. R., Choopanya, K., Vanichseni, S., & Ward, T.P. (1992). International epidemiology of HIV and AIDS among injecting drug users. *AIDS, 6*, 1053-1068.

Feinberg, M. (1996). Changing the natural history of HIV disease. *Lancet, 384*, 239-246.

Flaskerud, J.H. (1995a). Health promotion and disease prevention. In J.H. Flaskerud & P.J. Ungvarski (Eds.), *HIV/AIDS: A guide to nursing care* (3rd ed., pp. 30-63). Philadelphia: Saunders.

Flaskerud, J.H. (1995b). Psychosocial and psychiatric aspects. In J.H. Flaskerud & P.J. Ungvarski (Eds.), *HIV/AIDS: A guide to nursing care* (3rd ed., pp. 308-338). Philadelphia: Saunders.

Flaskerud, J.H., & Ungvarski, P.J. (Eds.). (1995). *HIV/AIDS: A guide to nursing care* (3rd ed.). Philadelphia: W.B. Saunders.

Grady, C., & Kelly, G. (1996). HIV vaccine development. *Nursing Clinics of North America, 31*, 25-39.

Grady, C., & Vogel, S. (1993). Laboratory methods for diagnosing and monitoring HIV infection. *Journal of the Association of Nurses in AIDS Care, 4*(2), 11-21.

Greene, W.C. (1997). Molecular insights into HIV-1 infection. In M.A. Sande & P.A. Volberding (Eds.), *The medical management of AIDS* (5th ed.). Philadelphia: Saunders.

Grimes, D.E., & Grimes, R.M. (1994). *AIDS and HIV infection.* St. Louis: Mosby.

Grimley, D.M., DiClemente, R.J., Prochaska, J.O., & Prochaska, G.E. (1995, Spring). Preventing adolescent pregnancy, STD and HIV: A promising new approach. *Florida Educator, 7-15.*

Haynes, B.F. (1996). HIV vaccines: Where we are and where we are going. *Lancet, 348,* 933- 927.

Health care worker occupational exposure to HIV. (1994). *International AIDS Society - USA Newsletter. 2*(1):1,19.

Ho, D., Neumann, A., Perelson, A., Chen, W., Leonard, J., & Markowitz, M. (1995). Rapid turnover of plasma virions and CD4+ lymphocytes in HIV-1 infection. *Nature, 373,* 123-126.

Hughes, M.D., Johnson, V.A., Hirsch, M.S., Bremer, J.W., Elbeik, T., Erice, A., Kuritzkes, D.R., Scott, W.A., Spector, S.A., Basgoz, N., Fischl, M.A., & D'Aquila, R.T. (1997). Monitoring plasma HIV-1 RNA levels in addition to CD4+ lymphocyte count improves assessment of antiretroviral therapeutic response. *Annals of Internal Medicine, 126,* 929-938.

Jadack. R.A., Hyde, J.S., & Keller, M.L. (1995). Gender and knowledge about HIV, risky sexual behavior, and safer sex. *Research in Nursing and Health, 18,* 313-324.

Johnston, M.I. (1997). HIV vaccines: Problems and prospects. *Hospital Practice, 32,* 125-138, 140.

Joint United Nations Programme on HIV/AIDS. (1997, December). Global summary of the HIV/AIDS epidemic. Available: http://www.unaids.org/highband/document/epidemio/report97.html

Jones, R.S., & Gelone, S.P. (1997). Antiretroviral drugs to fight AIDS. *Hospital Medicine, 33,* 40-42.

Kinsey, K.K. (1994). "But I know my man!" HIV/AIDS risk appraisal and heuristical reasoning patterns among childbearing women. *Holistic Nursing Practice, 8,* 79-88.

Klaus, B.D., & Grodesky, M.J. (1997). Assessing and enhancing compliance with antiretroviral therapy. *The Nurse Practitioner, 22*(4), 211-219.

Lauver, D., Armstrong, K., Marks, S., & Schwarz, S. (1995). HIV risk status and preventive behaviors among 17,619 women. *JOGGN, 24,* 33-39.

Leonard, V.W. (1994). A Heideggerian phenomenological perspective on the concept of person. In P. Benner (Ed.). *Interpretive phenomenology: Embodiment, caring, and ethics in health and illness.* Thousand Oaks, CA: Sage Publications.

Lisanti, P., & Zwolski, K. (1997). Understanding the devastation of AIDS. *American Journal of Nursing, 97,* 26-35.

Lurie, P. L., & Drucker, E. (1996). An opportunity lost: Estimating the number of HIV infections due to the U.S. failure to adopt a national needle exchange policy [Abstracts-On-Disk]. XI International Conference on AIDS.

Lurie, P., Reingold, A. L., Bowser, B., Chen, D., Foley, J., Guydish, J., Kahn, J. G., Lane, S., & Sorensen, J. (1993). *The public health impact of needle exchange programs in the United States and abroad* (vol. 1). San Francisco: University of California.

Mandelbrot, L. (1997). Timing of in utero HIV infection: Implications for prenatal diagnosis and management of pregnancy. *AIDS Patient Care and STDs, 11,* 139-147.

Martin, F.J. (1996). STEALTH liposome technology: An overview. *DOXIL Clinical Series, 1,* 1- 8.

Masci, J.R. (1996). *Outpatient management of HIV infection* (2nd ed.). St. Louis, MO: Mosby.

Mascola, J.R., McNeil, J.G., & Burke, D.S. (1994). AIDS vaccines: Are we ready for human efficacy trials? *Journal of the American Medical Association, 272,* 488-489.

McFarland, G.K., & McFarlane, E.A. (1993). *Nursing diagnosis and intervention: Planning for patient care* (2nd ed.). St. Louis, MO: Mosby.

McNicholl, J.M., Smith, D.K., Qari, S.H., & Hodge, T. (1997). Host genes and HIV: The role of the chemokine receptor gene CCR5 and its allele (Δ 32 CCR5). *Emerging Infectious Diseases, 3,* 261-271.

Mellors, J.W. (1996). Clinical implication of resistance and cross-resistance to HIV protease inhibitors. *Infectious Diseases in Medicine* (Suppl.), 32-38.

Messiah, A., Dart, T., Spencer, B.E., Warszawski, J., & the French national Survey on Sexual Behavior. (1997). Condom breakage and slippage in heterosexual intercourse: A French national survey. *American Journal of Public Health, 87,* 421-424.

Moore, R.D., & Bartlett, J.G. (1996). Combination antiretroviral therapy in HIV infection: An economic perspective. *PharmacoEconomics, 10,* 109-113.

National Institutes of Health (NIH). (1997). Report of the NIH panel to define principles of therapy in HIV infection. Available: http://www.hivatis.org

Normand, J., Vlahov, D., & Moses, L. E. (Eds.). (1995). *Preventing HIV transmission: The role of sterile needles and bleach.* Washington, D.C.: National Academy Press.

O'Brien, W.A., Hartigan, P.A., Daar, E.S., Simberkoff, M.S., & Hamilton, J.D. (1997). Changes in plasma HIV RNA levels and CD4+ lymphocyte counts predict both response to antiretroviral therapy and therapeutic failure. *Annals of Internal Medicine, 126,* 939-945.

Occupational exposure to bloodborne pathogens: Final rule. (1991, December 6). *Federal Register, 235,* 64175-64182.

Olfson, M., Hansell, S., & Boyer, C.A. (1997). Medication noncompliance. *New Directions for Mental Health, 73,* 39-49.

Panel on Clinical Practices for Treatment of HIV Infection. (1997, November 5). Guidelines for the use of antiretroviral agents in HIV-infected adults and adolescents. Available: http://www.hivatis.org

Porche, D.J. (1997). Postexposure prophylaxis after an occupational exposure to HIV. *Journal of the Association of Nurses in AIDS Care, 8,* 83-87.

Price, R.W. (1997). Management of the neurologic complications of HIV-1 infection and AIDS. In M.A. Sande & P.A. Volberding (Eds.), *The medical management of AIDS* (5th ed.). Philadelphia: Saunders.

Prochaska, J.O., Redding, C.A., Harlow, L.L., Rossi, J.S., & Velicer, W.F. (1994). The transtheoretical model of change and HIV prevention: A review. *Health Education Quarterly, 21*(4), 471-486.

Saag, M.S. (1997). Use of HIV viral load in clinical practice: Back to the future. *Annals of Internal Medicine, 126,* 983-985.

Seals, B.F. (1996). Viewpoint: The overlapping epidemics of violence and HIV. *Journal of the Association of Nurses in AIDS Care, 7,*91-93.

Selik, R.M., & Chu, S.Y. (1997). Years of potential life lost due to HIV infection in the United States. *AIDS, 11,* 1635-1639.

Sowell, R. L. (Ed.). (1997). Adherence issues in HIV therapeutics [Special issue]. *Journal of the Association of Nurses in AIDS Care, 8*(Supplement).

St. Louis, M.E., Kamenga, M., Brown, C., Nelson, A.M., Manzila, T., Batter, V., Behets, F., Kabagabo, U., Ryder, R.W., Oxtoby, M., Quinn, T., & Heyward, W.L. (1993). Risk for perinatal HIV-1 transmission according to maternal immunologic, virologic, and placental factors. *Journal of the American Medical Association, 269,* 2853-2859.

Staprans, S.I., & Feinberg, M.B. (1997). Natural history and immunopathogenesis of HIV-1 disease. In M.A. Sande & P.A. Volberding (Eds.), *The medical management of AIDS* (5th ed.). Philadelphia: Saunders.

Thomasma, D.C. (1994). Toward a new medical ethics: Implications for ethics in nursing. In P. Benner (Ed.). *Interpretive phenomenology: Embodiment, caring, and ethics in health and illness.* Thousand Oaks, CA: Sage Publications.

Thompson, J.M., McFarland, G.K., Hirsch, J.E., & Tucker, S.M. (Eds.). (1993). *Clinical nursing* (3rd ed.). St. Louis, MO: Mosby.

Thorne, S.C. (1993). *Negotiating health care: The social context of chronic illness.* Newbury Park: Sage Publications.

Tovo, P.A., DeMartino, M., Gabiano, C., Cappella, N., D'Elia, R., Loy, A., Plebani, A., Zuccotti, G.V., Dallacasa, P., Ferraris, G., Caselli, D., Fundaro, C., D'Argenio, P., Galli, L., Principi, N., Stegagno, M., Ruga, E., Palomba, E., & the Italian Register for HIV infection in children. (1992). Prognostic factors and survival in children with perinatal HIV-1 infection. *Lancet, 339,* 1249-1253.

Ungvarski, P.J. (1997). Update on HIV infection. *American Journal of Nursing, 97,* 44-52.

Whipple, B., & Scura, K.W. (1996). The overlooked epidemic: HIV in older adults. *American Journal of Nursing, 96*, 23-28.

Williams, A.B. (1997). New horizons: Antiretroviral therapy in 1997. *Journal of the Association of Nurses in AIDS Care, 8*, 26-38.

Wilson, B.A. (1997). Understanding strategies for treating HIV. *MEDSURG Nursing, 6*, 109-111.

Additional Bibliographical References

Bayer, R. (1989). *Private acts, social consequences: AIDS and the politics of public health.* New Brunswick, NJ: Rutgers University Press.

Bradley-Springer, L. (Guest Ed.). (1996). Education [Special issue]. *Journal of the Association of Nurses in AIDS Care,* 7 (Supplement).

Cameron, M.E. (1993). *Living with AIDS: Experiencing ethical problems.* Newbury Park, CA: Sage.

CDC Advisory Committee on Prevention of HIV infection. (1994, June). *External review of the CDC's HIV prevention strategies.* Atlanta, GA: U.S. Department of Health and Human Services, Public Health Services.

Clark, C.F. (1994). *AIDS and the arrows of pestilence.* Golden, CO: Fulcrum Publishing.

Corea, G. (1992). *The invisible epidemic: The story of women and AIDS.* New York: Collins Harper Publisher.

DiClemente, R.J., & Peterson, J.L. (Eds.). (1994). *Preventing AIDS: Theories and methods of behavioral interventions.* New York: Plenum Publishing Corp.

Glaser, E., & Palmer, L. (1991). *In the absence of angels.* New York: Berkeley Books.

Kreiger, N., & Margo, G. (Eds.). (1994). *AIDS: The politics of survival.* Amityville, NY: Baywood Publishing Co.

Kurth, A. (Ed.). (1993). *Until the cure: Caring for women with HIV.* New Haven, NJ: Yale University Press.

Mann, J., & Tarantola, D. (Eds.). (1996). *AIDS in the world II: Global dimensions, social roots, and responses.* New York: Oxford University Press.

Ropka, M. E., & Williams, A.B. (1998). *HIV nursing and symptom management.* Boston: Jones and Bartlett.

Sanford, J.P., Gilbert, D.N., Moellering, R.C., Jr., & Sande, M.A. (1997). *The Sanford guide to HIV/AIDS therapy* (6th ed.). Vienna, VA: Antimicrobial Therapy, Inc.

Shilts, R. (1993). *Conduct unbecoming: Gays and lesbians in the U.S. military.* New York: Fawcett Columbine.

Shilts, R. (1987). *And the band played on: Politics, people, and the AIDS epidemic.* New York: St. Martin's Press.

Sontag, S. (1989). *Illness as metaphor and AIDS and its metaphors.* New York: Anchor Books, Doubleday.

Ungvarski, P. (Guest Ed.). (1997). HIV disease: New frontiers and emerging challenges [Special issue]. *Journal of the Association of Nurses in AIDS Care,* 8 (4).

Valdieserre, R.O. (1994). *Gardening in clay: Reflections on AIDS.* Ithaca, NY: Cornell University Press.

Verghese, A. (1994). *My own country: A doctor's story of a town and its people in the age of AIDS.* New York: Simon and Schuster.

Warner, S.O. (1995). *The way we write now: Short stories from the AIDS crisis.* New York: Citadel Press.

Index

Index

A

B

C

D

M

N

O

P

R

SKIDMORE-ROTH PUBLISHING, INC.

400 Inverness Drive South, Suite 260, Englewood, CO 80112

Ph. 1-800-825-3150

Title	Code	ISBN #	Price	Qty
INSTANT INSTRUCTOR SERIES				
AIDS HIV, Bradley-Springer 1995	ADIN01	1-57930-010-0	$9.95	
Hemodialysis, Fowlds 1994	DLN01	1-56930-020-8	$9.95	
NURSING CARE PLANS SERIES				
Critical Care, Comer 1998	CNCP01	1-56930-035-6	$38.95	
Geriatric (2nd ed.), Jaffe 1996	GNCP02	1-56933-052-6	$38.95	
HIV/AIDS (2nd ed.), Bradley-Springer 1999	ADSC02	1-56930-097-6	$38.95	
Maternal-Infant, Luxner 1999	NCP01	1-56930-099-2	$38.95	
Oncology, Gale 1996	ONCP01	1-56930-004-6	$38.95	
Pediatric, (2nd ed.), Jaffe 1998	PNOP02	1-56930-057-7	$38.95	
SURVIVAL SERIES				
Geriatric Survival Handbook, Acello 1997	G8G001	1-56930-061-5	$35.95	
Nurse's Survival Handbook, Acello 1999	NSHB01	1-56930-040-2	$39.95	
Obstetric Survival Handbook, (2nd ed.), Masten 1998	OBHB02	1-56930-083-6	$35.95	
Paramedic Survival Handbook, Martin 1999	PSHB01	1-56930-090-9	$29.95	
Pediatric Nurse's Survival Guide, Rebeschi 1996	PNGD01	1-56930-018-6	$29.95	
NURSING/OTHER				
Body in Brief, (3rd ed.), Rayman 1997	BBRF03	1-56930-055-0	$39.95	
Diagnostic and Lab Cards, (3rd ed.), Skidmore-Roth 1998	DLC03	1-56930-065-8	$29.95	
Drug Comparison Handbook, (3rd ed.), Reilly 1998	DRUG03	1-56930-075-5	$39.95	
EMS Field Protocol Manual, Apfelbaum 1999	PEMS01	1-56930-091-7	$24.95	
Essential Laboratory Mathematics, Johnson & Timmons, 1997	ELM01	1-56930-056-9	$29.95	
Geriatric Long-Term Procedures & Treatments, (2nd ed.), Jaffe 1999	GLTP02	1-56930-072-0	$36.95	
Geriatric Nutrition and Diet (3rd ed.), Jaffe 1998	NUT03	1-56930-096-8	$25.95	
Handbook of Long-Term Care (2nd ed.), Vitale 1997	HLTC02	1-56930-058-5	$28.95	
Handbook for Nurse Assistants, (2nd ed.), Nurse Asst. Consort. 1997	HNA02	1-56930-059-3	$23.95	
I.C.U. Quick Reference (2nd ed.), Comer 1998	ICQU02	1-56930-071-2	$39.95	
Infection Control, Palmer 1996	INFO01	1-56930-051-8	$119.95	
Nursing Diagnosis Cards (2nd ed.), Weber 1997	NDC02	1-56930-060-7	$31.95	
Nurse's Trivia Calendar, Rayman	NTC	1-56930-xxx-x	$11.95	
OBRA (3rd ed.), Jaffe 1998	OBRA03	1-56930-047-x	$149.95	
OSHA Book (2nd ed.), Goodner 1997	OSHA	1-56930-069-0	$124.95	
Procedure Cards (3rd ed.), Jaffe 1996	PCCU03	1-56930-054-2	$24.95	

Title	Code	ISBN #	Price	Qty
NURSING/OTHER (continued)				
Pharmacy Tech, Reilly 1994	PHAR01	1-56930-005-4	$25.95	
Spanish for Medical Personnel, Meizel 1993	SPAN01	1-56930-001-1	$25.95	
OUTLINE SERIES				
Case Management, Ling 1999	CMO01	1-56930-080-1	$99.95	
Diabetes Outline, Barnwell 1995	DBOL01	1-56930-031-3	$23.95	
Fundamentals of Nursing Outline, Chin 1995	FUND01	1-56930-029-1	$23.95	
Geriatric Outline, Morice 1995	GER01	0-944132-90-1	$23.95	
Hemodynamic Monitoring Outline, Schactman 1995	HDMO01	1-56930-034-8	$23.95	
Critical and High Acuity Outline, (2nd ed.), Reynolds 1999	HATO02	1-56930-094-1	$23.95	
Med-Surgical Nursing Outline, (2nd ed.), Reynolds 1998	MSN02	1-56930-068-2	$23.95	
Obstetric Nursing Outline, (2nd ed.), Masten 1997	OBS02	1-56930-070-4	$23.95	
Pediatric Nursing Outline, (2nd ed.), Froese-Fretz et al 1998	PN02	1-56930-067-4	$23.95	
RN NCLEX REVIEW SERIES				
PN/VN Review Cards, (2nd ed.), Goodner	PNRC02	1-56930-008-9	$29.95	
RN Review Cards, (3rd ed.), Goodner 1999	RNRC03	1-56930-092-5	$35.95 (tnt)	

Name _____

Address _____

City _____ State _____ Zip _____

Phone (_____) _____

☐ VISA   ☐ MasterCard   ☐ American Express   ☐ Check/Money Order

Card # _____ Exp. Date _____

Signature (required) _____

Prices subject to change. Please add $6.95 each for postage and handling. Include your local sales tax.

MAIL OR FAX ORDER TO:
    SKIDMORE-ROTH PUBLISHING, INC.
    400 Inverness Drive South, Suite 260
    Englewood, Colorado 80112
    1-800-825-3150

Visit our website at: http://www.skidmore-roth.com